"Al Vernacchio has masterfully accomplished what good sexuality educators have attempted for so many years: he has created a work that is both a fun, easy read as well as a thorough and thoughtful guide."

—Don Dyson, PhD, associate professor, Center for Human Sexuality Studies, Widener University

"Al Vernacchio has written a wonderful book that includes numerous model answers and a new way to think about adolescent sexuality—as a force for good in life rather than simply a problem to be dealt with."

—Leslie M. Kantor, PhD, MPH, chair of the Department of Urban-Global Public Health at the Rutgers School of Public Health

"Vernacchio's no-blame, no-shame approach will inspire parents to drop their fears, judgments, and inhibitions in order to help their kids navigate the teen years."

—*Publishers Weekly*

"An engaging, much-needed new approach to teaching children about the human sexual experience."

—*Kirkus Reviews*

T0007951

for

goodness

sex

for goodness sex

A Sex-Positive Guide
to Raising Healthy,
Empowered Teens

Al Vernacchio

with Brooke Lea Foster

HARPER

NEW YORK • LONDON • TORONTO • SYDNEY

HARPER

FIRST HARPER WAVE EDITION PUBLISHED 2014.

FIRST HARPER PAPERBACKS EDITION PUBLISHED 2023.

The Library of Congress has catalogued the previous edition as follows:

Vernacchio, Al.

  For goodness sex : changing the way we talk to teens about sexuality, values, and health / Al Vernacchio, with Brooke Lea Foster.—First edition.

    pages cm

  ISBN 978-0-06-226951-5 (hardback)

  1. Sex education. 2. Sex instruction for teenagers. 3. Sexual ethics. 4. Teenagers—Sexual behavior. 5. Parent and teenager. I. Title.

  HQ56.V46 2014

  613.9071—dc23

                        2014019134

ISBN 978-0-06-325129-8 (pbk.)

23 24 25 26 27 LBC 5 4 3 2 1

To my students past and present, who bring meaning, purpose, and joy to my work, and to Michael, who brings meaning, purpose, and joy to my life

Contents

Contents

Preface to the 2023 Edition:
Ten Years Later . . .

Ten years ago, I was already deep into my career as a sexuality educator. A string of amazing opportunities culminated in the first edition of this book. Fast-forward to a few months ago, when an invitation came from my publisher to revise and update it.

To my high school students, ten years is forever, but to my almost sixty-year-old brain, the past ten years was a blip. I had to step back and ask: Do I have more to say? Has that much really changed since 2014?

The answer to both questions, clearly, was yes: I have more to say, a few things to correct, and lots to reinforce. And, yes, some important things have changed. I don't know how historians will talk about the past ten years, but there's a lot worthy of attention: the Trump administration; the explosion of the #MeToo and the Black Lives Matter movements; increased visibility and social acceptance of transgender, nonbinary, queer, and questioning individuals and communities; the COVID-19 pandemic; the Capitol insurrection; the ever-growing presence of Internet pornography; the overturning of Roe v. Wade; "Don't Say Gay" bills; and our widening political and cultural divide. Given all this, it was clear that the new edition of this book needed a few changes: nongendered pronouns throughout, a renewed commitment to diversity and nonbinary thinking, a revised chapter on sex and gender, a full chapter on pornography, and a new chapter on consent as a tool in preventing sexual violence.

Sexuality education doesn't exist in a vacuum. We can use it as a means to reinforce or to challenge dominant paradigms. For me, sexuality education is a form of social justice education. I believe that comprehensive, progressive sexuality education should make people (and therefore the world) more free, more loving, more open, and more accepting. Through our conversations with teens, we help create a world where social ills (everything from unplanned/unwanted pregnancies to racism) are reduced.

That means that sexuality education and our conversations about it have to be intersectional. They have to look at how factors such as: age, ability, gender, race, religion, sexual orientation, and socioeconomic status (just to name a few) intersect and interact. When sexuality education is not intersectional it likely only reinforces the power and privilege that already exist in our society. So, when talking about body image, for example, it's important to think about how ethnic, racial, and religious differences may impact how people view their bodies. When talking about abortion, it's essential to talk about the political and cultural barriers that interrupt its availability. When talking about pleasure, we need to acknowledge the sexism that has caused female pleasure to be valued less than male pleasure. When talking about pornography, we can also talk about how it may fetishize certain groups of people.

One of the things that has changed in the past decade—and you won't be surprised by this—is the amount of information that is available to young people today and the easy accessibility of that information. Technology in the classroom and at home has progressed to the point where the world is truly at young people's fingertips, even though young people's brains aren't necessarily equipped to handle that much information. They need help discerning what information will actually be helpful to them and what will lead them into trouble. Our job today, whether as educators or parents, entails talking more about media literacy, about how to assess the validity of information, and about looking at the sources of information and their biases and values. Teenagers today likely don't need us to tell them how sperm cells form or what sexual intercourse is, but they do need help figuring out how to access that information and to determine what information exists for their benefit and what is trying to steer them away from authenticity and truth.

Another thing that's changed over the past decade is the process of identity formation. Whether we think this is a positive change or not, young people today have many more options to consider than simply whether they feel like a boy or a girl, and whether they are gay, straight, or bisexual. Our understanding of both gender identity and sexual/romantic orientation has greatly expanded over the past ten years, and we have an ever-increasing list of labels one can use to describe oneself.

To me, this is a great benefit because it allows young people to find a more precise way to describe their own experience. What it has also brought about is greater latitude in experimenting with different identities. It's not uncommon today for young people to try out different labels, different pronouns, and different relationships in search of their truth. This can be quite jarring for adults who had fewer options and were taught that identity, once established, was unchanging. I've had a lot of talks with parents and caregivers over the past decade about how it's perfectly normal for teens, and even younger kids, to shift how they think of themselves and how they label themselves. Yes, there certainly still are people who establish an identity early in life and don't shift, but the possibility of changes in both language and behavior is not uncommon today and shouldn't be looked at as a sign of confusion or a problem.

Yet, amidst all this, being a teen is still being a teen. Humans have pretty consistent developmental needs and go through developmental phases that don't seem to be radically affected by time or social tumult. I'm always amazed at how my students have the same questions year after year. This is actually good news for educators and adults who want to help kids. We can predict what needs a young person has and we get the chance to work at serving those needs more and more successfully as time passes. I'm a much better teacher of teenagers than I was ten years ago because I've had ten more years of practice working with them. I feel for parents and caregivers who often only get one or two chances to work through raising a teenager. Over the years at my school, almost four hundred students have taken my Sexuality and Society class. That's four hundred amazing, unique, funny, frustrating, charming, fumbling, and brave kids. How privileged I feel to be able to have so many opportunities to try to be a helpful presence in young people's lives.

Good sexuality education is age appropriate, medically accurate, value explicit, honest, joyful, intersectional, communal, and accessible to all learners. It's a natural extension of the education necessary to be a positive, helpful member of society. It's both intellectual and affective; there is a body of knowledge to be learned, but also time must be spent processing the emotions that may arise in learning this information. Emphasis should be placed on how to make a decision that is in accordance with one's values, and how to handle value conflicts. Ultimately, good sexuality education teaches us who we are most authentically and allows us to form relationships (both sexual and nonsexual) based in that authenticity and use those relationships to better the larger world.

You're reading this book because you care about young people and their healthy development. I do too. Together—me in the classroom and you in ordinary moments of your lives—we can support young people's growth and help them thrive. If the last decade has taught us anything it's that we need the hope, energy, and power of young people to help right the ship of this fractured and teetering world. Thanks for committing to that journey with me.

Introduction to the 2014 Edition:
Sexuality as a Force for Good

People often ask me, "What do you think of the state of sex in America today?" I always quote my friend Jeanmarie, who says that we're "sexually repressed to the point of being sexually obsessed." Let that sink in a bit because it's the best description I have for how we treat sexuality in this country. We are a nation founded by people who saw sex as something sinful, and this sex-negative view has followed us all the way to the twenty-first century. It's made us into a society that's incredibly uptight and uncomfortable when it comes to talking openly about sex. Yet when we flip through *Vogue* and come across a racy Dolce & Gabbana ad or find ourselves engrossed in *Fifty Shades of Grey*, we're as titillated by our interest as we are disgusted by it.

Sexuality education today typically falls into one of two categories. "There is abstinence-only sex education, and there's abstinence-based sex ed," Leslie Kantor, vice president of education for Planned Parenthood Federation of America, told the *New York Times*. "There's almost nothing else left in public schools." When the HIV/AIDS epidemic broke out in the early eighties, there was a steady stream of funding for programs teaching safer sex. But most of that funding went to "abstinence education," which aimed to keep teenagers from having any sexual activity at all, largely by limiting information to the most basic biological facts and relying on fear-based tactics that highlighted the dangers of sex. Some of you probably remember an abstinence-education video that was often shown in classrooms in the 1980s and '90s called *No Second Chances*. In the film, a teenager asks a school nurse, "What if I want to have sex before I get married?" The nurse responds, "Well, I guess you'll just have to be prepared to die."

In 2011, President Obama gutted the budget for abstinence-only education, in part because there's no evidence that it stops kids from engaging in sexual intercourse. According to a government report, prepared by Representative Henry A. Waxman, many abstinence-only programs also taught scientific inaccuracies about sex. *The Waxman Report* notes that one federally funded program passed out materials that said that HIV/AIDS could pass through a condom because the latex is so porous, which experts say isn't true.* Sexuality educators today can be so stifled by school boards that, according to the *New York Times Magazine*, some are asked in job interviews if they can teach sex ed without saying the word *sex*. Both abstinence-based and abstinence-only approaches rely on "disaster prevention," meaning that educators are presenting sex and its consequences as dangerous, potentially catastrophic events. Sex can kill you or ruin your life.

Is that really what sex is to us? It's not what it is to me, and I doubt that's what sex is to you. But how can we possibly expect young people to go from those scary, sex-negative messages to establishing relationships based on trust, intimacy, and pleasure?

....

* *The Content of Federally Funded Abstinence-Only Education Programs*, United States House of Representatives Committee Government Reform—Minority Staff Special Investigations Division, December 2004.

How *can* you have a good sexual relationship when no one ever tells you how to do that? There's plenty of talk about what *not* to do, but that doesn't automatically provide a road map for creating a happy and successful sexual life.

It's the silence from the trusted adults in their lives that leads so many kids to go to the Internet for answers. If you Google "what is oral sex," "fingering," or "falling in love," you get millions of hits, and many of them are from sources you *wouldn't* want your kids to trust. It's likely your child will click from one pornographic site to the next in search of an explanation that could have been provided by you in a few sentences. The types of images they see online are bound to give them an unhealthy view of gender and sexual activity. Unfortunately, we're living in a world where Internet pornography is the basic template that many kids use to define what sex is like, what they're expected to do physically in a relationship, and how they're supposed to look when they're doing it.

Chances are that if you're not talking to your kids about sex, their sexual education is more like a junk food diet; they're picking up whatever they can from movies, commercials, TV, video games, and online porn. That's why I strive so hard in my classes to help kids see themselves accurately—as sexual beings who have values and choices to make, as authentic individuals with a set of likes and dislikes, as real people who aren't *supposed* to look like models on billboards or porn stars in movies. I teach them not to make sexual decisions based on how attractive or unattractive they think they are. I ask them to examine their gender identity and sexual orientation and understand the impact they have on their sexual activity.

I can't imagine standing up in front of a class of twenty seniors—

young fresh-faced kids getting ready to go off to college—and telling them that having sex is going to ruin their lives. How does that help them develop healthy sexuality? What kind of message would I be sending about intimacy, love, and relationships? Instead, what if we equipped our children to know and love their bodies, to see their partners as unique individuals rather than sex toys, and to make decisions based on accurate information and their own values? What if we sent kids off into the world with a clear view of the role that sexuality plays in their lives, now and for years to come?

Rather than just telling them what's *not* OK, what if we worked at telling them what *is* OK? Notice I haven't talked penetration. I haven't mentioned semen. I won't go there in my class until we get to a place where we're all ready. Teaching kids about sexuality is about giving them the skills, the framework, for putting themselves out there in the world with confidence. It's about valuing healthy bodies and healthy minds. It's about giving young people the tools to make healthy choices.

Here's what you need to know about me: I'm an educator. I've wanted to be a teacher since I was five years old (except for a brief stint in fourth grade when I wanted to be the pope). I'm not a therapist or a clinician. I'm not a parent, although as a teacher for almost thirty years, I've certainly acted in a parental role to countless kids. I'm also not just some creepy old guy who likes to talk about sex. I have a master's degree in human sexuality education from the University of Pennsylvania. I was drawn to my work, in part, because I've always been able to talk openly and easily about sex. I always quip that when God was passing out talents, I got ease in talking about sex. So let's get to it.

CHAPTER 1

Teaching Healthy Sex

On the first day of my Sexuality and Society class, I don't pass around anatomy drawings. I don't hand out pamphlets about safer sex, although those are stacked on a table near the door. Instead, the first thing I do is establish ground rules. I do this while standing at my podium at the front of the class in my sweater vest and tie, a wall of buttons and pins behind me. Some of my favorites say: RESIST HOMOPHOBIA, FIGHT SEXISM, ENJOY LIFE. THIS IS NOT A DRESS REHEARSAL, and TEACH, DON'T BULLY! I'm all about context. Talking about sexuality, intimacy, relationships, and pleasure can't be done in a vacuum. So we establish guidelines: people should speak for themselves, laughter is OK, we won't ask "personal history" questions, and we'll work to create a community of peers who care about and respect one another. Only then can we get to work.

One of the early activities in class involves handing out blank index cards to the students and asking them to write down the first thing that comes to their mind when they hear the word *sexuality*. I tell them that I'm going to collect the cards, shuffle them, and read their responses aloud. This affords them safety to say what they really think and to hear their peers' responses anonymously.

Many of the cards say things like, "sex," "having sex," or "being straight, gay, or bi." Some of the cards say, "relationships" or "hooking up." Some are blank, while others say, "I really don't know; nobody's ever asked me that before."

They're not bad definitions, and they already reveal a certain amount of vulnerability, which will grow as the course continues. "Those are all good answers," I tell them. "But isn't sexuality more personal than that? Isn't it about knowing yourself as much as it is about engaging in anything physical?" At the beginning of the year, I'm always reminded of how young teenagers are, despite how old they try to act, and how little they actually know about sexuality, or even their own bodies.

I like to challenge kids to think about sexuality as a philosophy, not an act. Over the course of my time with them, I'll focus on the positive role that healthy sexuality can play in their lives.

I decided a long time ago that my role as a sexuality educator isn't to get teenagers to have or not to have sex—that's something they'll decide as they grow to know themselves and their values more clearly. But I do see it as my job to get kids to think more thoughtfully about sexuality, to learn what it means to respect their bodies, and to offer them a positive and realistic framework from which to make sexual decisions. I do this by staging dialogues about love and relationships, gender roles in high school and in society, how we choose personal morals and values, and sexual orientation. I give them a chance to ask questions, even taboo ones, by slipping a piece of paper into the class Question

Box or posting a question anonymously on the class blog. I've gotten questions that range from "How do you know you're in love?" to "Are you a semi-virgin if you've had oral sex but not intercourse?" to "How can I love my body more?" to "Do people from different races make different-colored sperm?"

As we start to talk about what sexuality is, I hand out a worksheet that asks students to rate how they feel about different aspects of themselves—their bodies, their emotional selves, their gender, their spiritual selves. They can choose from ratings like "love it," "feel OK about it," and "don't like it." A girl in skinny jeans and a high ponytail marks "love it" for her mind, "don't like it" for her body. When the students are finished, I call them back to attention.

"So, there's a lot more to this than just sex, isn't there," I say. "Sexuality is the way our our bodies, gender, and sexual orientation influence how we act in the world and the way the world reacts to us. Healthy sexuality means having an accurate and positive view of ourselves, and using that as a basis for our relationships and our life choices."

They look . . . confused, so I continue. "We're not just walking genitals, right?" They laugh, and I laugh along with them. "We're whole people with bodies, brains, emotions, and spirits. All of those things are part of our sexuality. When we interact with the world, we do it with these bodies we carry around with us. We filter the world through our gender (agender, woman, man, genderqueer, nonbinary, etc.). We also look at the world through the lens of our sexual orientation (asexual, straight, queer, demisexual, pansexual, etc.)—whom we are attracted to and whom we fall in love with. All of those things are involved as we make decisions about what to do with our genitals, aren't they?"

The boy in the corner wearing sweatpants and a hoodie says, "I guess, but how?"

"Well, take me, for example," I say. "I'm a short, fat, hairy, white, Italian American man. I'm gay, and have been with my husband for almost thirty years. I'm a person who laughs a lot and leads with my heart rather than my head. Spirituality and religious faith are essential parts of my life. Do you think all those things affect how I behave in the world, including in my sexual life? Do you think they influence how the world sees me and reacts to me?"

"Aww, Mr. V," a girl pipes up and gives me a big smile. "You're not fat."

"Fat, plump, round, fleshy—call it whatever you want," I say, smiling back at her. "I'm still sexy as hell."

The class erupts into hoots and hollers.

"But go back to my question. Do you think my body, my gender, sexual orientation, physical appearance, temperament— all those things I just listed about myself—have an impact on my actions and the world's reactions to me?"

"Yeah, sure," says a boy with shaggy blond hair and glasses. "What does that have to do with my sexuality?"

"Those are all the things that make up *my* sexuality," I say, clapping my hands.

Now I know I've got them interested. They're thinking about sexuality—they're even *talking* about sexuality, and we're not talking about intercourse. Not yet.

....

What comes to mind when you think about the words *teens* and *sex*? If you're like most of the population, you might have thought:

"teen pregnancy," "condom," "HIV," or "STD" (sexually transmitted disease, which you might also see referred to as STI, sexually transmitted infection). So much of how we see a young person's sexuality is defined by all of the things that can go wrong. Parents work hard at being there for their children in every way. They try to make every soccer game and pay for expensive SAT prep courses; they check in with their kids via text all day long and offer to drive car pools. But for many sane, logical, really good parents, talking about sexuality is fraught with anxiety. It's avoided or handled in a one-time "pat on the back" talk. Many parents tell me that they're relieved I'm talking with their kids about sex because then they don't have to. I understand that perspective, but disabuse them of the idea quickly. Yes, to talk about sex with our kids makes us vulnerable, which is not the role we're used to playing in our kids' lives. And many parents will say that their kids would rather die than talk to them about their relationships. Guess what? You have to talk to them anyway.

I agree 100 percent with the idea that parents must be the primary sexuality educators of their children. I know that teens *want* their parents to talk to them about sex. Your kids might make a big, loud production out of telling you to go away or to stop talking, but don't be fooled. They're listening. They want to know what it means to be in love with someone, why senior guys often want to date freshman girls, what to do when you *can't stop thinking about someone*. And they want to know how their parents handled all of these things. Have you told your child the story of your first kiss? Have you shared stories of crushes you had as a teen and how you handled them? Have you told them how you knew you were in love with your sweetheart, or how you managed your first big breakup? Whether you did these things well or not isn't the point. Kids learn as much, maybe more, from hearing about our failures as they do from hearing about our successes. We don't owe kids perfection, just humanity.

Let's think for a moment how challenging it is to be a teenage boy: One day you're a sweet little kid flying your superhero action figures around the living room, and then out of nowhere, you're riding the Hormone Express! Your feet shoot out like a clown's, your voice begins cracking when you talk, and your armpits start to stink. You've already seen naked bodies on the Internet—whether you intentionally went looking for them or stumbled onto them by accident—but now you want to see *real* naked bodies, in person, and the thought alone can send you into a tizzy. Walking to the front of the classroom to conjugate a Spanish verb or standing in the lunch line carries the intense fear that you're going to get a sudden erection, especially when you're, say, carrying your lunch tray and can't hide it easily. I've been teaching ninth-grade boys for decades. At the beginning of the year, they're like tiny puppies that can barely keep from peeing on the rug. By the end of the year, they're tall and deep-voiced. They're growing into young men.

Teenage girls come into ninth grade generally feeling more confident than their male peers. They know that they're physically and emotionally more mature than the boys their age; their bodies started their own wild ride back in middle school. But soon these same girls are beating themselves up for not being pretty enough or skinny enough. They may dress to accentuate their new curves, but then may feel conflicted about the attention they get from wearing low-cut shirts or short skirts. They worry about coming off as too smart in class. They see the way women are portrayed in the media and it both attracts and repulses them. They see Lizzo loudly and proudly loving her big body and wonder if they should lean into that idea or run from it. They fear being called a slut while at the same time they're being told that slut-shaming is bad. It can all feel like a lose-lose proposition. And they *feel* all these things deeply, as well as emotions like attraction, lust, and love. Yet when asked, many of them can't actually define what any of those words mean.

And what about the kids who identify as nonbinary, agender, gender fluid, or genderqueer? They have language to define themselves, but painfully few role models who can teach them what it means to live outside the realm of binary gender. On the plus side, these kids are excellent at critiquing our society's antiquated and stifling gender expectations, but on the minus side, they are often forced to explain or speak on behalf of all nonbinary individuals and may lack adult champions who see, understand, and nurture them. Often they have to rely on each other for support and protection from adults who do them more harm than good.

I'm not saying these things to scare you or encourage you to lock up your children in the basement until they are thirty, despite how much you may want to. I know you love your children, and you want the best for them. So do I. Seeing your children as sexual beings is a very difficult thing for many parents to do, considering you're still doing their laundry, buying their underwear, and laying out a spread of snacks during sleepovers. But many of your kids are going to engage in sexual activity whether you want to imagine it or not.

In addition to my twelfth-grade class, I also teach a human

sexuality class to the ninth-graders at my school. Before the course started, I gave each of my twelfth-grade students a card and asked them to write down a piece of advice they wished someone would have told them when they were in ninth grade. "Wait for the right time," one student wrote. Another said, "Don't be pressured to have sex." One girl wrote, "Don't let people make you feel bad about yourself." Kids grow a lot during high school, and nowhere is this better shown than in these wise notes from my older students. They illustrate just how overwhelming the topic of sex is for many kids and how much good advice they can give each other when given the chance.

I'm just about the least likely person you'd expect kids to ask their most important questions about sex. I'm a short, round, gay guy rapidly approaching sixty. I am not what Hollywood would call attractive or sexy. And yet, for many kids, I'm the only sounding board they have. They know that when they ask a question in class or come to see me privately with a question about sex, I will not panic, avert my eyes from theirs, fake an answer, or find a reason to put on the TV. Apparently, that's what a lot of parents do, according to my students. It's also what my parents did. Kids will try to ask a question about sex—"What age did you lose your virginity, Mom?" "Is Dad the only person you've ever been with?" Parents get so nervous at being ambushed with a sex talk that they stumble over their words and avoid answering the question. The kids walk away feeling more confused than before they asked, and many will avoid asking their parents a sex question again.

I know parents don't always feel equipped to answer these questions, especially when they're sprung on them unexpectedly. That's one of the reasons I wanted to write this book. I want you to see that you *can* have these conversations with your kids, and I'll give you some concrete ways to do it. You don't need to have your own master's degree in human sexuality education; you just need to be an honest, authentic person who wants the best for your child. That's the same message I give your kids when they come to talk with me. Start from honesty, lean into trust, and believe that sexuality is a force for good. From there, it's a piece of cake—really!

....

The first step is learning to see our own kids' sexuality as a *necessary and normal* part of the human lifespan from birth to death. We are born with bodies, emotions, and desires—including sexual desires. Forming connections with other people is essential to our survival as babies; in fact, the first, and most important, intimate relationship healthy children develop is with their parents. Breastfeeding is one of the most important expressions of healthy sexuality a mother and baby can experience. It doesn't start from a place of sexual arousal or seek to produce sexual pleasure, but it's a powerful expression of healthy sexuality. Our children were given bodies for many reasons, one of which was to make them feel safe and good and connected to others. As adolescents it's healthy for them to want to be with another person. It's normal for them to want to kiss that person, write them a love note, and even make a decision about how much of their body they want to share with that person. They're going to look in the mirror and stare and grimace and pose. These are all age-appropriate thoughts and actions that emerge in the teenage years.

It's important to remember that when I talk about kids (or

any persons) as sexual beings, I don't necessarily mean sexually *active* beings. Those are two different things. If you're not OK with thinking about your children as sexual beings, let's figure out why. One reason is that your parents probably didn't raise you to think of yourselves as sexual beings. How many of us get messages early in our lives about loving our bodies, about pleasure being an important and healthy part of life? Did your parents see sexuality as a force for good in the universe? Until we can get rid of the old programming that tells us sex is sinful or dirty or dangerous, it'll be hard to celebrate healthy sexuality in our kids.

Another reason these beliefs can be hard for us is that when we look back on our own teen years, we're much more likely to remember the things that went wrong than the things that went right. We remember the shame, heartache, and pain of our own adolescence. We don't want our kids ever to feel that way; we hope that's a part of life our kids *don't* experience. And even if we remember experiences that were thrilling and wonderful, we're not quite sure it's OK to tell our kids about them.

But why not? We need to talk about all of those experiences— the good and the bad, the agony and the ecstasy. Healthy sexuality doesn't mean our kids will never experience heartache or regret or make a mistake. Of course they will. They're human. Here's the thing, though: When we made those mistakes, were there adults in our lives who could help us process them without blaming or shaming? Did anyone help us to put our choices and experiences into context? Did anyone help us think through what we really wanted and why, and how to maximize the chance that we'd find the good and minimize the chance we'd get hurt? Probably not. But what if we can do that for the young people in our lives? That starts the day we can see them positively as sexual beings on their way to adulthood.

Once you can accept that your child is a sexual being, you're one step closer to being able to talk to your kids about their sexuality. And that also involves setting limits for them. Right now your kids need guidance in knowing what is OK to do, what's OK to consider doing, and what just isn't OK. Fear-based threats don't lead to positive behavior change, so can you begin to consider a more open dialogue with your kids around these ideas?* For example, your fourteen-year-old might say they're in love. But stop before you say something like, "That's ridiculous. You don't know what love is yet." What if you used the opportunity to have a conversation about what fourteen-year-old love looks like? In a situation like this, I might say, "Tell me what that feels like. It's been a long time since I felt love as a fourteen-year-old." I might also say, "Isn't it great to kiss and hug and hold someone you love?"

Many kids become sexually active with each other because they don't know what else to do. In movies, everyone jumps to sex, so they assume that's what they're working up to as well. I've had kids ask me: "What do you do if you love somebody?"

"You make them food," I say.

They'll giggle, like you probably did. But you can go on to make your point: there are many different ways to show someone that you love them.

....

* B. L. Frederickson, "What Good Are Positive Emotions?" *Review of General Psychology* 2, no. 3 (1998): 300–19; Gerard Hastings, Martine Stead, and John Webb, "Fear Appeals in Social Marketing: Strategic and Ethical Reasons for Concern," *Psychology and Marketing* 21, no. 11 (2004): 961–86.

What if our kids could turn to us for information, for guidance, for assurance that they're OK? What if they could grow up with a critical eye able to see through the unhealthy messages they get each day? What if they believed they were worthy of love *and* pleasure, just as they are? This really can happen for our kids, but the first step is for us to see them as fully sexual people and to believe that their sexuality can be the force that leads them to true happiness, not hedonism or heresy.

As we take this journey together through the book, I urge you to keep your eyes on the prize—young people who know their values, who believe themselves worthy of love, who feel good about their bodies, who see pleasure as a means to build intimacy and connection with another, and who live their lives not fearing mistakes but using them as lessons to reorient themselves toward success. Impossible, you think? I've seen it happen year after year with my students—and I'm just their teacher. Think about how much more amazing they will be when their parents believe this too.

....

Question Box

When I started teaching human sexuality I kept an old shoebox with a hole cut into the top of it in my classroom. Next to the box were slips of paper and pencils. Kids could place anonymous questions in the box for me to answer in class. These days the Question Box has gone high tech. There's a link on my class web page where kids can submit their anonymous questions. The old shoebox is still in the classroom, but it's more a relic now than a functional tool.

At the end of each chapter, I'll include some actual questions from students and my answers to them. I haven't done any fancy editing of the questions or answers. I'm including the actual questions as kids asked them and my unedited responses to them. I do this for a couple of reasons. First, I want you to see what kind of questions kids are actually asking. They run the gamut from innocent to downright technical. I also want to model answering these questions, to show you how I approach a topic and how even a simple question allows for both information and value clarification to be offered in response. So here are a few general questions from the box to get us started:

Q: Why is sex so good?

A: There are two ways to answer this question. From the biological perspective, sex feels good for an important evolutionary reason. If a species, like ours, is going to reproduce sexually, then there's an advantage if that action also feels good. As I've often said, if sex felt like getting your tooth drilled at the dentist, people wouldn't have it very often, and that could eventually threaten the survival of our species. Our bodies have evolved so that our genital regions, as well as many, many other parts of the body, are sensitive to sexual stimulation. A part of the body that brings sexual pleasure when stimulated is called an *erogenous zone*. This does not mean just our genitals. All of us have many places on our bodies that result in sexual pleasure when stimulated. Knowing your own and your partner's erogenous zones can lead to much more fulfilling sexual experiences. The mechanisms of sexual pleasure involve a combination of nerve impulses, blood flow, and muscle tension. To find out more about this, you might

Google the phrase "human sexual response cycle" and look at the work of Masters and Johnson, two famous sex researchers who studied the body changes that happen when people get sexually excited.

The second reason sex feels good is that humans have developed the emotional capacity to feel love, intimacy, and passion. These emotional states highlight and deepen sexual pleasure. While pleasure can exist without these emotions, it is much more significant when they are present.

Q: When is someone emotionally and physically ready for sex?

A: I wish I had an answer that would be right for all people at all times, but the real answer is "It depends." We are all unique individuals, and our relationships are all unique. Because of that, there can't be a standard answer to this question. Wouldn't it be great if we could say, "The Thursday following your sixth date is the most appropriate day to start having sex"? But, of course, that's not the way it works.

I think it's appropriate to start being sexually active with a sweetheart (and remember: I define *sexually active* as being involved with someone else's body for the purpose of giving and receiving sexual pleasure) when intimacy, commitment, and passion are established and both people have pretty equal amounts of these feelings for each other. I don't think these things develop quickly, so I don't think sexual activity is appropriate on a first date or early in a new relationship. I also think people aren't ready to become sexually active if they can't talk about it with their partners in a serious way, and also talk about safer sex practices, contraception (if appropriate), and possible positive and negative consequences and how they'd deal with them. Emotionally, a person has to be ready to face other people's responses, positive or negative, to the sexual activity and be willing to share those emotional reactions with his or her partner.

As you can see, I think it takes a lot for a couple to be ready to engage in sexual activity. If any of the above things aren't in place, I'd say you're not ready.

Q: Could you use a balloon as a condom?
A: Short Answer—ABSOLUTELY NOT!!! UNSAFE! UNHEALTHY! DANGER! DANGER!

Longer Answer: OK, I'm calmer now. Condoms are made to be condoms; balloons are made to be balloons. Both can be made of latex, but that doesn't mean they're interchangeable. You wouldn't use a pencil eraser as a car tire even though they're both made of rubber, would you?

Condoms, when used correctly, are an essential tool in reducing the risk of pregnancy and STIs. They work so well because they're designed for that purpose. No condom substitute (balloon, plastic baggie, sock—whatever) will provide the same level of protection, and some can do more harm than good. So insist on the original! Sometimes people ask about condom substitutes because they don't know where to get condoms or are embarrassed to get them. Condoms can be purchased at any local drugstore; there are no age requirements for buying condoms and no prescriptions are necessary. Free condoms are available from many health clinics, sexual health agencies, and even some schools (although ours does not provide free condoms at this time).

Here's an important thing to consider. If a person doesn't feel confident enough to acquire condoms, then maybe they shouldn't be having intercourse. Being ready for sexual intercourse means being able to handle all aspects of the situation, including protecting oneself and one's sweetheart from unwanted consequences. Remember my rule about sexual activity—"If you can't look your partner in the eye and talk about it, then you can't do it with them." My rule for condoms is, "If you can't take responsibility for securing condoms, then you're not allowed to have the kind of sexual activity that calls for using condoms."

Q: How can you tell if a guy likes you?

A: I know you're really hoping for a clear-cut answer here, but that's just not the way it works, I'm afraid. People can react in all kinds of ways when they like you. Some people get really quiet around you. Others will make sure you notice them. Some will tease you or act annoying. Some will just silently stare at you (yes, that can feel a little creepy).

The best way to figure out if a guy likes you is to *ask him!* Might it feel awkward to do that? Sure, but it's also a way to get a clear answer. You might want to resort to the middle school tactic of asking your friends to ask his friends if he really likes you or not, but that makes the whole thing so much more public than it needs to be. You could try using Facebook or texts to figure it out, but they're not great ways to get clear information.

Why not try the kind of "I message" we use in class? In an I message, you describe the situation, say what you feel, and say what you want or need. Below are two different I messages you might try (or make up your own!).

#1: *"I'm trying to figure something out and I could use your help. I'm feeling a bit confused about what you think of me. I'm wondering, can you be honest with me and tell me whether you like me or not?"*

#2: *"It's hard for me to figure out if someone likes me or not. I'd be a lot less anxious if I knew for sure. So, I was just wondering, do you like me?"*

Asking such a question might seem scary, but remember, the worst a person can say is no, and you're absolutely strong enough to hear that and be OK. Believe it! Then go ask him.

CHAPTER 2

Creating a Family Philosophy of Sex: What We Believe, What We Say, and How We Say It

As my students file into class on a late-winter day, happy to escape the chill outside, they look up at the board and smile. Two boys high-five. A voice I'm not meant to hear whispers, *Finally!* On the board I've written, "What is having sex?"

We weren't ready to talk about this until now. In a sexuality education classroom, as in any healthy relationship, intimacy and trust don't just happen. They need to be developed. Only after talking about the basic definition of sexuality, about values and language, about our bodies, and about gender as both a biological and social construct are we ready to move on to the topic of sexual activity. We know each other; we've practiced listening to one another; we've had our first few awkward and heated discussions. We can handle this now.

What they don't realize is that we're also about to have another conversation about values.

As I begin the class, I ask students for their definitions of the phrase *having sex*. In the beginning of the year, I would have asked them to jot down their definitions on index cards, but at this point in the semester, they're ready to shout out answers uninhibitedly. There's a variety of responses, as usual, everything from slang ("two people doing it") to comedic ("shakin', bakin', and makin'") to technical ("penis inserted into the vagina"). Someone shouts, "Home run!" No matter the group, someone always shouts, "Home run!"

"Let's think about this in a bit more detail," I say, passing around a handout. It contains a long list of possible sexual behaviors. I tell the students, "Go down the list and put a check mark next to anything that you think would be having sex. Then look at what you've selected and summarize that into a definition of having sex." The noise level in the room increases. "Do this on your own, please," I say. "You need to know what *your* definition is, and your friends can't tell you that."

After they've completed the activity, I ask for a volunteer to share the definition.

A young woman in a long floral skirt pipes up. "Vaginal intercourse that leads to orgasm in one or both partners." As I write the definition on the board, I smile, because they think we're finished, but we've just gotten started.

"OK, does anyone want to add to that definition or alter it?"

"Just a penis," someone asks, "or can it be vaginal penetration with a sex toy or a finger?"

"No! Just a penis—duh!" one of the boys shouts.

"So, is it the penis or the penetration that makes it having sex?" I ask.

Voices erupt all over the classroom.

"It's the penis!"

"Maybe a sex toy but not a finger!"

"That's sex but not *real* sex!"

"Gotta be a penis!"

"What about anal?"

"Ewwwwwwww!"

"But, wait, then lesbians can't have sex?"

As our discussion, and sometimes our debate, continues, I revise the definition on the board. Often we wind up with multiple definitions. Some are more inclusive, some less. Some include an emotional component, others only mechanical acts. As I draw this part of the lesson to a close, I ask a series of questions that prompt the class to think about not just *how* they define having sex, but also *why*.

"Think about these things," I say. "How do your values about orgasm influence your definition of having sex? How do your values about the primacy of genitals versus other body parts influence it? How do your values about gender and sexual orientation influence your definition? What effect do your values about relationships or love have on your definition of sex?"

Over the years, this activity has evolved. Now, I tend to focus more on the conditions and qualities necessary to have healthy sex than on what behaviors are being done. In fact, when I give the students my definition of healthy sex there are no behaviors specified. I define healthy sex as "consensual, sober, safer, sexual activity that offers mutual pleasure, intimacy, and enhanced connection." I have to be honest—the kids hate this definition. They're totally on board with consensual, but they balk at sober (even though they know that drunk sex is terribly unsafe for lots of reasons). They question whether sex has to be mutually plea-surable and whether it has to bring connection and intimacy. A frustrated young man, one of the ones who high-fived his friend at the start of the class said, "I don't wanna talk about values! I wanna talk about having sex!"

"You can't talk about one without the other," I say, smiling.

....

Over my many years as a sexuality educator, I've found that people are more afraid of talking about their values than about their sexual activity. Many people aren't even sure what a value is, and they've certainly never taken a deliberate inventory of their values around sexuality. My students are like this when they appear in my class. They're eager to start talking about the ins and outs of sex, pardon the pun, and when they hear we're starting with the topic of values, they look completely flummoxed.

There are many different theoretical frameworks for talking about values. I have been most influenced by the work of Sidney B. Simon, Leland Howe, and Howard Kirschenbaum and their clas-sic text *Values Clarification*. I use their ideas as the basis for my teaching about values. A simple definition of the term *values* is: the deepest-set rules that guide one's decisions. Values don't just tell us *what* we do; they tell us *why* we do it, which is much more important. Our values reflect our core beliefs; they tell us what really matters to us. Most people strive to do what they think is right or correct in any given moment or circumstance. Your values help to guide each of those seemingly separate decisions, helping you determine what's right in an ethical, moral, or spiritual sense.

There are two immediate traps that must be avoided when

talking about values. The first is the idea that a choice or action can be "value free" or "value neutral." My students love to try to argue these positions when I present them with a "what if" situation or a dilemma to solve. But it's an argument they can't win, because *every* choice is based on one or more values; it's just a matter of figuring out what value is at work. One who consistently makes choices by flipping a coin values chance. One who decides things haphazardly, without a lot of thought, values chaos or impulsivity. Every academic subject in school is based upon a set of values. Math and science are based upon the values of logic, linear thinking, and order, and history rests on the value of a record of the past for insightful lessons and as context for making decisions in the present. Every school has its own code of values (which might be called school philosophy or mission statement). Every family has a set of values by which it operates. It's essential to clarify what values are at work for an individual or group before talking about sexuality.

The second trap in talking about values is the misunderstanding that they are relative. My students are always trying to answer a values question with "It depends," but they know it's an answer I don't accept. In my opinion, values relativism is just a cover for the value that's really at work—sometimes it might be selfishness or narcissism, other times it might be fear of being different. I think values relativism is used as an excuse to escape responsibility for our choices, for being too scared to admit what our values really are, or for simply being too lazy to really figure out what values are at work in a given situation.

It's essential when talking about values, and especially important in sexuality education, to distinguish between a fact, an opinion, and a value. A fact is something indisputable. Facts are sometimes argued, but they can be proved true with verifiable evidence. An opinion is a view or judgment formed about something—a fact, an event, a belief, a comment, anything. Opinions don't always rest on a sound foundation. They can be informed or uninformed. They can be based on fact, supposition, emotion, or even pure speculation. They can be defendable or not. My students often think that their opinions should reign supreme—after all, it's how they *feel* about something—but only by understanding the process used to form an opinion can we tell whether or not it's worth anything. A value, as defined above, is a core belief that guides actions and decisions. It has more emotional resonance than an opinion, and is often felt with zealous conviction, but it's not a fact. A value answers the "why" question at the deepest level.

To make these distinctions more clear, let's look at a few examples:

Fact: 2 + 2 = 4

Opinion: Math is hard!

Value: Proficiency in computational skills is essential for a successful life.

Fact: Washington, DC, is the capital of the United States.

Opinion: Capitals should be the largest city in a state.

Value: Representational democracy should ensure equal access to all.

Fact: Same-sex marriage is legal in some states.

Opinion: Same-sex couples should have some legal rights but not the right to marry.

Value: The heterosexual family unit is the most valuable grouping in society.

In his book *Values and Teaching*, Louis Raths explores what he calls *valuing*, a process by which we can determine whether an idea is really one of our values or not. First, a value must be chosen freely from alternatives after careful consideration of its consequences. It cannot be something thrust upon us or adopted without significant forethought. Second, a value must be prized and publicly affirmed when appropriate. If we're ashamed of it, won't talk about it, or won't defend it to others when called upon to do so, it isn't a value. Third, and to my mind most important, a value must be acted upon consistently and repeatedly. If we say it but don't do it, it's not a value. If we follow it sometimes but not consistently, it's not a value. It is only by understanding what our values really are that we can make sense of our choices. It's also important to remember that values are aspirational. While we may strive to live according to our values all the time, we fail to do this simply because we are human. Guilt often results when we do something that goes against one of our values. But rather than letting guilt get the better of us and cause us to feel shame, we can use the feeling of guilt to our advantage, as a gentle reminder of what's truly important to us. It can be a useful tool if we reframe it. While we will not be able to live up to our values in every moment of our lives, we should continually strive to make choices that support our values in every area of our lives.

Values are both personal and societal. There are countless

institutions that offer values they think we should adopt as our own. Parents and families, schools, religious organizations, governments, media, and peers are just some of the groups that present us with rules for living. As adults we usually affiliate ourselves with groups and organizations that share our core values. I choose to teach at a school that espouses the values I hold dear. It's a small private school founded by the Religious Society of Friends, also known as the Quakers. Its bedrock beliefs include simplicity, peace, integrity, community, equality, and stewardship. But children seldom get to choose their early values or sources of values. They are born into families, sent to schools, brought to worship services, and bombarded with many forms of media. They are offered many different sets of values each day and, as they grow, must begin to make choices about which speak truth to them.

Because we may adopt different values from different sources, value conflicts often emerge. Common conflicts for adolescents involve family values versus those offered by peers or media, the value of immediate gratification versus planning for future consequences, and the value of self-interest versus the interests of others. Value conflicts are useful for helping us to determine what's really most important to us, and sometimes the answers are not what we expect.

There is an activity at the end of this chapter called Twenty Things I Love to Do, which I use in class to help students begin to discover their values. It's taken from *Values Clarification*, although I've tweaked it a bit. This is an activity you can do yourself or with your teenager. My students always find it enlightening. I hope you will too.

Valuing Sexuality

Once you complete the Twenty Things I Love to Do activity, you'll notice that, although you completed the phrase "I love to" twenty times, you didn't uncover twenty different values. Most people don't have a laundry list of values to suit every activity or situation. In fact, having a lengthy values list is a sign, to me, that someone hasn't really determined his or her core values. That's not the way values work. Because they are the foundation upon which we build our lives, we generally have a small set of core values that continually guide our actions and find expression in a number of different areas of life. So it's not that we have separate sexual values, political values, spiritual values, etc. We have values that express themselves in all of those areas, and those expressions should be consistent across those different areas. So as we begin to talk about sexual values, it's important to keep in mind that most are expressions of more deep-seated values.

It's also important to consider if our basic attitude toward sexuality leans toward positive or negative. Most people aren't exclusively at either end of the spectrum, but neither are they exactly in the middle. Some people view sexuality as a fundamentally dangerous force. They see it as dirty or wild, and believe that if unrestrained, it can lead to lives of wanton hedonism. Others may have a negative orientation toward sexuality because of past incidents of abuse or sexual trauma. As you can see by the title of this book, my fundamental value about sexuality is that it is good. One of my most important mantras is "Sexuality is a good gift from a good God." I see sexuality as the force that allows us to be our most authentic, loving, and connected; it's the best thing about being human. That may be a hard thing to believe for a person who is a survivor of sexual abuse or trauma, and I respect that. I'm not saying everyone has to have a positive orientation toward sexuality. I'm saying it's important for each of us to look inward and see what our basic orientation toward sexuality is, to understand how that influences the decisions we make, and to become aware of the ways in which that orientation is expressed to our children. My positive orientation toward sexuality doesn't mean that I have an "anything goes" attitude. In fact, because I believe sexuality is a force for good, my guidelines for behavior, whether in the classroom, in my relationships, or in life in general, are actually quite stringent. Doing the thing that brings about the most authentic and loving result isn't always doing the easiest thing. It doesn't allow for selfishness, disregard of others, or falseness.

For example, here are different guidelines about sexual activity that can result from different core values:

- Sexual activity should be about love more than about sex.
- Pleasure should be the guiding principle in sexual activity.
- If I can get it, I'll take it.
- In sexual activity, what I want matters less than what my partner wants.
- Safety is more important than pleasure.
- If my religion says it's OK, then it's OK.
- If I can tell my parents about it without feeling ashamed, then it's OK.

Now think about the last few months of your life and any decisions you've made that involved sexuality. This can be anything from how you answered a question your children asked to what you chose to watch on television. Do those decisions seem in line with the core values you identified above? Think about the way that social media has become such a seemingly essential part of life. That required a huge shift in societal values. Our values about communication, intimacy, and privacy have all been affected. Have we taken the time to think about that, or have we just adopted these new values uncritically? Or think about what happens when your child is headed out to a party dressed in clothing you think is inappropriate, or when your four-year-old decides to take off his or her clothes in the supermarket. Nudity, abortion, masturbation, sexting, privacy, body image, pornography, contraception, and even love: all of these topics will surface at some point with our children. If we want to help them navigate choices about these things, we're going to be a lot more successful if we know how our core values affect them and if we can help our kids think about *their* values and the impact they have on *their* behavior.

One of my core values is equity, which is different from equality. Equality says give everyone the same thing. This sounds like a great idea, until we realize that we don't all start out in the same place. Equality does not necessarily correct for injustice; in fact, it may perpetuate it. Equity asks us to give people what they need so that everyone can achieve the same outcome. In order to achieve pleasure equity, for example, some people might need more time, permission, stimulation, or lubrication than others in order to achieve an amount of pleasure we would say is desirable in a sexual encounter. Because I value community over individuality,

I think discussions about sexuality with others are valuable, instructive, and healthy. Because I do not value selfishness, I can't condone sexual activity or relationships wherein only one party has access to pleasure or orgasm.

It's essential for parents to talk with their children at every age about values. What are the family values that they are expected to abide by? Where are they free to determine their own values? What sources of values does the family consider to be especially important and which sources does the family reject? For example, do the values of your child's school match your family values and, if not, where might they diverge? We do not always have the luxury of sending our children to schools that perfectly reflect our family values. So what do you say to your child when he or she comes home confused after learning at school that homosexuality is wrong, but they don't see anything wrong with Uncle Joe and Uncle Jim who are a part of your family?

In the same way that parents make and display lists of chores for their children, it can be useful to have a list of the family's core values displayed in a common area where they can be referenced and discussed. Making family values explicit is the best way to create ongoing dialogue and clear expectations for children and teens.

Helping our children develop a strong value system can certainly contribute to healthy sexuality. Of course we want to guide our children in the process of creating a value system, and we should be involved, but a moralizing approach—"Do it because I say so"—doesn't work.

Instead, I'd urge an approach in which an individual can freely choose his or her own values based upon guidance from trusted sources, exploration, information, careful consideration, and experience—what Simon, Howe, and Kirschenbaum call "value clarification." In moralizing, the goal is to instill the parents' values in their children. Value clarification, though, seeks to have a person develop a set of values that are *uniquely their own and defendable.*

A Word About Language

OK, so you're starting to feel more prepared to have a conversation with your child or teen about sexual values. But how do you start? What language should you use? How can you increase the chance that your message will get through without your adolescent rolling his eyes or stomping out of the room? After all, talking about sexual values and sexuality in general can be difficult even with your peers (or your spouse!) because, as the old Gloria Estefan song says, "Words Get in the Way."

I think the words get in the way because people believe that there's a "right way" to talk about sexuality, but that's not true. There are many different paths to a successful conversation because there are many different languages of sexuality. Being multilingual and knowing which language will work in a given situation is the key.

In order to help my students understand the different languages of sexuality, I do a classic sex-ed activity. I put large sheets of paper around the room. At the top of each sheet is a term or phrase related to human sexuality. I ask my class to come up with as many different ways to say that term or phrase as they can, using words and phrases they've heard, read, or possibly used. The only rule is that they can't invent new terms or phrases. The words at the top of the pages are *penis*, *vulva/vagina*, *breasts*, *masturbation*, *sexual intercourse*, *homosexual/heterosexual*, and *foot* (yes, the thing at the end of your leg). The students are timid at first, wondering whether they'll get into trouble for writing down some of the language they use with each other. With encouragement from me, they loosen up and the room erupts into noise, laughter, applause, and sometimes disagreement. After they've exhausted their store of alternate language, we bring the sheets to the front of the room and display them prominently on the board. I always make the kids laugh by saying, "Just think how proud your parents would be! Look at all the cool words you know!" I add that I'll post the sheets in the classroom on parents' night. Some students assume I'm joking and laugh, while others look worried because they think I'm serious.

A few things become apparent just from scanning the lists. There are lots of aggressive or threatening words for *penis*: spear, shaft, snake, rod, pecker, drill, gat (a machine gun). Words for *vulva/vagina* are either floral sounding ("rosebud") or nasty ("nappy dugout," "axe wound")—there's very little in between. There are lots of words for *breasts*, but how many of them are used to describe male breasts? Why are female breasts sexualized but not male breasts? Likewise, the words and phrases for *masturbation* are almost exclusively male-oriented, although we know people of all genders pleasure themselves. Words for *intercourse* focus on penile-vaginal intercourse; almost no one considers oral sex to be intercourse, even though Merriam-Webster's definition of intercourse is "physical sexual contact between individuals that involves the genitalia of at least one person." The *homosexual* side of the sheet overflows with alternative words and phrases, almost exclusively derogatory or demeaning, while the heterosexual side is largely blank, usually listing only "straight" and "normal." And then there's *foot*. Although there are alternate words for foot ("dogs," "boats," "wheels," and "piggies" or "tootsies" for *toes*), students often have a hard time coming up with any of them. Why is that? It's because no child ever got smacked or scolded for saying *foot* out loud in public. The activity quickly shows the reason for all our euphemisms for sexual terminology: many people think they're dirty words. That also reveals something important about people's values around sexuality, doesn't it?

After that initial process, we spend the rest of the class discovering and differentiating the many languages of sexuality that appear on the lists.

Slang is the first language we discuss. While some people think slang is synonymous with crude or dirty talk, the Merriam-Webster definition is "language peculiar to a particular group," or "an informal, nonstandard vocabulary." Slang varies in its usefulness because it differs according to time, place, culture, orientation, and age—sometimes it needs translation. When I was growing up in South Philadelphia in the 1970s and '80s, if you said you "dated" someone, that meant you French-kissed them, not that you went out on a date with them (that was called "going out"). "Hook up" is a great example of modern sexual slang. Its definition can vary from "meeting up with someone" to "making out" to "having intercourse with." If you hear your kids talking about their friends "hooking up," don't assume you know what it means—ask them, and realize it may mean different things in different contexts. Slang has its uses, but it isn't the best language choice for parents who want to have conversations with their kids. Nothing will clear a room of teenagers faster than a parent trying to use sexual slang.

Secret language is pervasive in discussions about sexuality. This is language whose meaning is intentionally kept obscured or unexplained, or something shared only confidentially with a few. While everyone who hears it may not understand slang, it's not a secret. This language is different because it's intended to obscure. In every generation, young people create a secret language to talk about sex without adults catching on or butting in. A few years ago, middle schoolers would talk about the "pen15" club. "Pen15" was secret language for penis. It's great language if you're in on the secret but can be dicey if you're not. When I was in eighth grade, a lot of the other boys would ask me if I had "done it" yet. They were asking whether I'd gotten sexual with a girl yet, but I didn't know that. I didn't have any idea what "done it" meant, but I knew the right answer to their question. "Sure, I've done it!" I said with all the bravado of a preteen boy. "I did it last week and I'm gonna do it again tomorrow." Of course, that was enough to convince them that I hadn't done it and that I didn't know what "done it" meant.

Sometimes secret language is used to cover up the discomfort of the speaker. It's frequently used this way in discussions about sexuality. When we talk with children about their "private parts" or refer to a vulva as "down there" or use any of the euphemisms for a period ("my friend," "the curse," "her monthly," "a visit from auntie") we're using secret language and are likely missing out on an opportunity to have an important conversation about sexuality. When my mom wanted to have a "sex talk" with me, her own discomfort with discussing anything sexual led her to use secret language. She sat me down at the kitchen table one day when I was thirteen or fourteen and told me we should have a talk about "the marriage act." She said as I was growing up I would become more interested in "the marriage act." It was natural to be curious about it, and she said that "the marriage act" was a beautiful thing when used properly, but it was only for married people—that's why it was called "the marriage act." She asked me if I had any questions. The question I most wanted to ask was, "What the hell is the marriage act?" Instead, I shook my head no and got as far away from the kitchen table as I could. Of course, she was referring to sexual intercourse, but it would be a couple of years before I figured that out. I already knew what intercourse was by the time I was thirteen, but there was no way I could connect it to Mom's "marriage act." I look back on this encounter with sadness today. My mom was trying to be a good parent, to convey to me information as well as a value framework for sexual intercourse, but because she was uncomfortable, she resorted to secret language. The resulting conversation was awkward, short-lived, and never repeated.

And in the years since then, I've learned that even "correct" terminology can be interpreted as secret language if the audience isn't familiar with the terms used. Years ago I was the Volunteer Coordinator and Trainer for Philadelphia's largest AIDS-service organization. Part of my job was to conduct AIDS education programs in the community. I had just finished a workshop in which I discussed how HIV is transmitted and how "safer sex practices" could minimize the risk of transmission when a young man approached me with a question. He didn't want to ask it during the presentation because he was embarrassed, but he didn't know what I meant when I kept saying "safer sex practices." He actually thought I was saying "save for sex practices." He wasn't sure if he should be saving money or sperm or what. I felt like a complete idiot. There I was, confident that I was providing useful, correct, factual information about HIV, but I was speaking a secret language and this young man missed one of the most important parts of the presentation. When I clarified that by "safer sex practices" I meant things like knowing one's own HIV status, using a condom or other barrier protection during sexual activity, and limiting one's number of sexual partners, he said, "Oh, I've been doing all that. So I guess I've saved myself with my save for sex practices." This time I wrote out the phrase "safer sex practices" on a piece of paper and showed it to him. "Oh," he said, "that makes a lot more sense." We talked for a few more minutes as I gently tried to figure out if I'd screwed up anything else in the presentation.

There is language we create specifically to talk to small children about sexuality. There are many childlike words for little kids' genitals (*wee-wee*, *coochie*, *pee place*). If we talk about sexual activity at all with children, we say things like "making babies" or "Mommy and Daddy's special hug" rather than "having sex." Or we don't talk about it at all. I remember being in the bathtub around age six and pointing to my testicles.

"What are these?" I asked my mother.

"You'll need those later," she responded.

"Then why do I have them now?" I asked. But that was the end of the conversation.

Children pick up on the fact that there are certain body parts we use special language for or don't talk about at all, and because they don't understand why, they can develop shame, fear, or confusion about their genitals or about sexuality in general. There's no reason that a child who knows the words *elbow*, *ear*, and *leg* shouldn't also know the word *penis* or *vulva*. "But what if they say it *out loud*, in front of other people?" some parents will ask me with a hint of horror in their voice. What *is* wrong with that besides being potentially embarrassing for the adults in the room? I've also seen adult children talking to their parents about sexuality and still using childhood language. They never found a way to replace that language with something else around their parents. Believe me, that sounds far more ridiculous than a three-year-old saying *penis*. My professional and personal opinion is that there's no need for childhood language. It only leads to more difficult conversations down the road.

A very important and often ignored sexual language is romance language. The best example that comes up in the classroom exercise is "make love" for *intercourse*. Do we ever intentionally teach young people how to talk about sex or about their sweethearts in a loving, romantic way? Early in the year I introduce the term *sweetheart* as my regular term for a romantic (and possibly sexual) partner. I say things like, "When you and your sweetheart are trying to figure out what to do on the weekend . . ." or "What do you suppose a sweetheart might think about that?" Of course the term *sweetheart* doesn't apply in every instance, and that's an important lesson too. A hookup is not a sweetheart. Here's another example of romance language. There's a big difference between saying something "arouses" you versus something "gets you wet." Calling someone your "lover" is certainly a different message than referring to your "lay." We need to help young people think and speak in ways that convey the passion, love, intimacy, and commitment that can exist in a relationship.

There's also some very old sexual language that still hangs on in our vocabulary today. Words like *wedlock*, *maidenhead* (for hymen), and *deflower* (for losing one's virginity) are just a couple of examples. This archaic language is often sexist, heterosexist, and sex-negative. Can't you just imagine a character on *Downton Abbey* talking about performing her "wifely duties" (a common Victorian euphemism for sex)? We might find archaic language interesting from a historical perspective, but it doesn't have any place in contemporary discussions about sexuality.

Finally, there's medical or biological language. These are the words printed on the top of the large paper sheets in my classroom. This is the standard language for classroom sexuality education, medicine, academia, and formal discussions of sexuality. Just like all the other languages, though, it isn't appropriate in every situation. I'm not sure a sweetheart is longing to hear, "Let's have sexual intercourse tonight, darling." And friends chatting casually about sex may find it more appropriate to use slang or shared secret language. But the biological language can be a great one for parents and children to use together, with two caveats. First, although perfectly appropriate, a lot of people feel ashamed to use even these words. They need to be deshamed if you're going to use them with your kids. If they pick up on your embarrassment or hesitancy in using the language, they might also feel that you're ashamed of sex. We need to be empowered to use this language and to empower others to use it as well.

In preparation for your talk with your child or teen, why not practice saying the words out loud in front of a mirror? You can also practice the words with a friend or your spouse before springing them on the kids. The second caveat is to make sure you actually know the proper words and their usage. I've met too many people who call a vulva (a female's external genitals) a vagina (which is an internal organ). When my dad gave me his version of the "sex talk," he had a problem with the words. He called me into my parents' bedroom one evening when I was about fifteen. I thought I was in trouble or that someone had died; those were the typical reasons for being summoned there. Instead my dad said, "It's time we had a talk about . . . mastication." I thought I had misheard him. I was sure he was talking about masturbation and not chewing, but he continued. "Lots of boys your age masticate—that's normal. But you can't masticate too much. And you don't want to think dirty things about girls when you masticate. You have to respect women." I sat there biting the insides of my cheeks so I wouldn't laugh at Pop, who was really trying his best. Should I have used that as a teachable moment to gently and lovingly let him know the difference between the words *masticate* and *masturbate*? I was fifteen, grossly embarrassed, and still not sure I wasn't in trouble, so I did what most teenagers did. I said "OK, Pop. Thanks," and got the hell out of there. I must admit that, although hilarious, this was not a bizarre moment in our house; Pop was famous for mixing up words. My favorite was when he called the gas pedal in the car the "exhilarator" instead of the "accelerator." "Get your foot off the damn exhilarator!" he would yell at me when I was learning to drive. "You trying to kill us?"

We must be fluent in all of these languages of sexuality in order to be the most effective communicators we can be. The key is using the language that will be most appropriate for a given situation. None of these languages are wrong all of the time, and none of them are right all of the time.

A Few Conversation Starters

If you haven't yet had a conversation with your kids about values, language, or sexuality, you're probably feeling a little anxious about approaching the topic. That's normal; your kids are nervous too, although probably less than you are. It's natural for the first conversation to be a little bumpy. After all, you're trying something new. You can't expect to be an expert right out of the box. Isn't that what you'd tell your child if she or he was about to try something new? It's a good idea to practice ahead of time, visualize how you want the conversation to go, and maybe even test-drive it with your adult children or a close friend.

It can also be helpful to remember that these conversations don't need to be long to be effective. One of my favorite sexuality educators Deborah Roffman says it's always better to have one hundred one-minute talks than to have one one-hundred-minute talk.

Although the first conversation might be a bit awkward, talking about sex doesn't *have* to feel that way. One of my favorite lines when I talk with parents is, "Talking about sex with your kids is no different than talking about anything else . . . no matter how much you want it to be." "Clean up your room." "You're never too old to kiss your mother." "I love you." "Condoms are a must if you have intercourse." All of these sentences can be spoken the same way, and more important, all of them can be heard the same way—as loving (and slightly annoying) parental wisdom, and they all take less than a minute to say!

The best conversations about values and sexuality are triggered naturally. A news story on TV, a song on the radio, an ad in a magazine, a TikTok—all can be used to start a conversation. Dialogue about sexual values is more successful when it flows naturally into and out of conversation than when we create separate moments for "serious talks." Don't think you can have a verbal conversation? How about texting "Have a great day at school, and remember that consent is sexy" to your teen? Or how about a lunchbox note that says, "Your body is beautiful just as it is!" Maybe you'll leave a note on the desk in your kid's room or on their bed. The goal is to get a face-to-face conversation going, but getting your message across in any way is a definite win.

If you want to start a verbal conversation but you don't know how, here are a few opening lines to try:

"Since you're mature enough to drive / have a cell phone / make your own bed (whatever), I think you're mature enough to talk with me about . . ."

"I know we haven't talked much about sex before, but it's been on my mind lately. So, can I ask you something?" (Or "can I tell you something?")

"Can I tell you a wish I made for you last night? I was thinking about what a great kid you are and how much I love you, and I wished that you . . ."

"Have you heard that new song (insert title here)? Are the kids at school listening to that? I thought it was pretty gross, the way it talked about women. Do you hear that when you listen to it?"

"Did I ever tell you about the first boyfriend I had, when I was

sixteen? He was so cute that I actually blushed whenever he looked at me. . . ."

See, it's easy. I'm not going to let you off the hook when it comes to talking with your kids about values and sexuality. Throughout this book I'll be offering lots of information, examples, and practical advice for talking to your kids, or any kid you love, about healthy sexuality. They need us to do this. Remember, the conversation is already happening. Your kids are talking about sex all the time. It's just a matter of whether or not you join the conversation.

....

Question Box

Q: Is it bad to give oral sex to a girl?

A: First, let's clarify what we mean by a sexual activity being "good" or "bad." This definition can come from many different sources. Here are three things I think about when determining whether something is good or bad:

VALUES: A good sexual activity is one that follows our core values about sex, pleasure, relationships, etc. A bad sexual activity is one that violates our values.

INFORMATION: A good sexual activity is one that proceeds from accurate information about the act and its potential positive and negative consequences. A bad sexual activity is one based on mythology, rumor, or speculation.

CONSENT: A good sexual activity is one in which all parties involved freely and knowingly consent to the activity. A bad sexual activity is one that is performed without the consent of the parties involved or when the ability to consent is compromised through something like pressure or substance abuse.

Given these ideas, I would think it's bad to give oral sex to a girl if it violates a person's values of what sex should be, if a person is not well informed about what performing oral sex means or the consequences, or if it is done without consent.

Perhaps your question is more about the potential risks associated with giving oral sex to a girl. While there is no risk of pregnancy with oral sex, there is risk of STI transmission. If a woman is infected with an STI, her vaginal fluids can transmit that infection (either through the mucous membranes that line the mouth or directly into the bloodstream if there are any cuts or open sores in the mouth). Oral sex carries a lower risk of STI transmission than vaginal or anal intercourse, but the risk is there. Using a dental dam when performing oral sex on a woman reduces the risk of STI transmission. Besides the potential physical consequences, there are possible emotional consequences of oral sex. It is essential to make sure both parties are prepared for the intimacy and emotional connection that oral sex may bring.

Q: When is masturbation harmful?

A: Let's answer this question in two ways—physically and emotionally.

Physically, there are no harmful effects of masturbation. I guess a person could masturbate so frequently as to make the genitals sore. In that case, I hope the person would have the sense to stop and give the body a chance to heal and rest a bit. But in terms of harmful physical effects on fertility, sexual performance, sexual desire, or anything like that, there aren't any.

On the emotional side, if masturbation makes people feel guilty, ashamed, or in any way negative about their bodies or themselves, then I think they might consider not doing it while they try to work on those issues. It is possible to work through negative feelings and change the way you think and react, but if masturbation really violates someone's core values, then I'd advise them not to do it. It's certainly not healthy to do something deliberately to yourself that brings you physical or emotional pain.

I'd also say that masturbation becomes harmful when it isolates us and takes the place of human-to-human interaction. If someone would consistently rather stay home and masturbate than go out with friends, I think that's a problem. Anything that isolates us from others and locks us away from healthy connections with the world has to be examined.

Q: Is having sex with a person you just met a bad thing if you've talked to them about it?

A: You've heard me say in class that because I value personal connection, intimacy, and openness, my rule for any kind of sexual activity is, "If you can't look your partner in the eye and talk about it, you shouldn't be doing it with them." But that doesn't mean being able to talk to them is the *only* thing that gives a green light to sexual activity.

When people say they "just met," it's important to clarify whether they mean they literally never saw each other before this moment or they mean they kind of know each other but hadn't actually talked or had a lot of contact before now. It's *not* OK to have any kind of sexual contact with someone who's truly a stranger. That's dangerous and is an absolute NO! in my book. If it's a person who goes to the same school as a friend and has been seen around before but this is the first personal contact, that might be a different story. Even in that case, though, my personal opinion is that having any kind of penetrative sexual activity (oral, vaginal, anal) isn't OK with *any* person one has just met, even if you've talked about it. In terms of making out (kissing and touching), it's still a no in my book for a stranger and a maybe with a person someone's known about but having contact with for the first time.

I also think it matters where two people "just met." To my mind, there's a big difference between meeting a person at a party where there may be alcohol or other substances in use and meeting a person in the library while studying for a *Macbeth* test. Context matters, and I think people have to take that into account when making a decision.

Finally, there's talking and then there's *talking*. Saying to someone at a party, "You're cute. Let's hook up" isn't what I mean when I say two people should talk before getting sexual with each other. It's got to be talking that establishes some kind of real connection. That kind of talking includes clearly conveying positive, active consent, which is essential for any sexual contact in my book.

That's a long answer to your question, but I hope the information helps you clarify your own values and make a decision that's healthy for you and for the other person.

TWENTY THINGS I LOVE TO DO

I Love to . . .

	A	FR	FA	NS	FS	$	PR	ER	UN	C	TS
1)											
2)											
3)											
4)											
5)											
6)											
7)											
8)											
9)											
10)											
11)											
12)											
13)											
14)											
15)											
16)											
17)											
18)											
19)											
20)											

INSTRUCTIONS:

1. Complete the phrase "I love to . . ." twenty times, one in each box following the number. Note that these are things you

love to *do*, not things you love in general. Your answers can be specific ("I love to get ice cream with my grandpa") or more general ("I love to eat ice cream"). The answers should cover as many different aspects of your life as possible.

2. After listing the twenty things you love to do, go to each vertical column and put a check mark in the box if it applies to that thing you love to do. For example, in the first column put a check mark next to anything you prefer to do alone. You *can* have multiple check marks next to any item.

A = things you prefer to do alone

FR = things you prefer to do with friends

FA = things you prefer to do with family

N5 = things that would *not* have been on your list 5 years ago

F5 = things you think will *not* be on your list 5 years in the future

$ = things that cost *you* more than $5.00 to do every time you do them

PR = things that carry physical risk when doing them (you can define what physical risk means)

ER = things that carry emotional risk when doing them (you can define what emotional risk means)

UN = things you do that make you unconventional

C = things you hope will be on your children's list when they do this activity

T5 = pick the top five things you love to do from the list and number them 1 (highest) through 5 (lowest)

3. After checking off each of the columns, look at your results and think about the following questions. You might journal about them or discuss them with a trusted person.

What did this exercise confirm about your values?
Did anything from this exercise surprise you about your values? What?
Is there anything you might want to change about your values given the results of this activity? Why or why not?
With whom would you be willing to share this sheet? What does that say about your values?

CHAPTER 3

Baseball, You're Out!
Sexual Activity Without the Bases

One morning after the students have filed in and settled down, I ask them, "If I said that we were going to play ball today, what would you say?" There are giggles and smiles and some murmuring.

"What kind of ball are we playing?" asks one of my more rambunctious boys.

"How about baseball?" I say with a smile. "Batter up!"

"Do you mean baseball or *baseball*?" he asks.

I play along. "What do you mean? Are there different kinds of baseball?"

"You know there are," he says, playing right back. "And I'm good at both of them."

"Pretty good at rounding the bases and scoring runs?" I ask.

"Well, I don't want to brag," he says, "but when you've got the right bat the magic happens." Some of the other boys in the room break into peals of laughter. Some of the girls snort in derision.

"Are you going to let him get away with that?" I ask, looking around at the young women in the room who have challenged this boy before.

"It's OK, Mr. V," one of them says with a grin. "I have a feeling he won't be scoring anytime soon." The class erupts into roars of laughter and shouts of protest.

"OK, OK," I say, tying to reestablish some semblance of order. "We seem to have slid from baseball right into sex. Funny how that happens, isn't it?"

"I see what you did there, Mr. V," says the boy who started this off. Of course he does. I wasn't trying that hard to be subtle.

I launch into my lesson for the day. "Isn't it true that if you talk about sex with people, it's common to wind up talking about baseball? And even if people aren't using baseball language, isn't it true that when people think of sex they think about it like baseball?"

....

It seems that America's favorite pastime isn't just a sport—the baseball model represents our country's take on what it means to have sex. The problem is that it is seriously flawed, yet many people invoke the metaphor every day without really giving thought to the larger implications of the words they're using. Think about some of the more benign models we use in our everyday lives. For instance, most of us have a morning routine. There's an order to the way you start your day. For some, it might be: make coffee, shower, brush teeth, get dressed. For others, it might be: shower, make coffee, get dressed, brush teeth. These tasks are typically performed without much thought and they follow a pattern that's repeated (and reinforced) each time.

I call these routine ways of doing things *conceptual models*. Models help us understand rules, expectations, and procedures. Once internalized, models can have a powerful influence on the way we think and behave—they influence our everyday habits and routines. For example, when it comes to getting dressed, any number of models can produce successful results. We probably don't think about the fact that there might be more than one model, but when we find ourselves, as I do, with a husband who thinks that pants go on before socks when in my model socks go on before pants (*obviously!*), those models become crystal clear. Models for dressing are benign, but a problematic model that gets internalized can lead to unhealthy outcomes. The "sex is like baseball" metaphor has become a conceptual model in our culture; it's certainly the basic framework for the way most young people learn about sex from their peers, and it has an impact on their habits and behaviors. For example, in a heterosexual interaction, a girl might make a rule for herself about what base she'll allow a boy to "go to" on a first date. It's an arbitrary rule and may have little to do with her own values, wants, and needs, but it's derived from widespread acceptance of this conceptual model. The baseball model also provides the standard language used for talking about sex in the media and in popular culture. Unfortunately, it's hugely problematic.

One of the ways we know that baseball has become an internalized model for sexual activity is by how casually we invoke this metaphor. Want a few examples? I've got plenty! First, there are the "bases," which refer to specific sexual activities that happen in a very specific order and ultimately result in "scoring a run" or "hitting a home run." This usually means having heterosexual vaginal intercourse to the point of orgasm, at least for the guy (there's one glaring problem with the model). People are generally "pitchers" or "catchers" and that corresponds to whether you perform a sexual act or receive a sexual act. You can "strike out," which means you don't get to have any sexual activity. If you're a "benchwarmer," you might be a virgin or somebody who isn't "in the game"—maybe because of your age or because of your ability or your skill set. A "bat" is a penis, and a "nappy dugout" is a vulva or a vagina. A "glove" or a "catcher's mitt" is a condom. A "switch-hitter" is a bisexual person, and those in the gay and lesbian community "play for the other team." And there's this one: "If there's grass on the field, play ball." That means if a young person—specifically a young woman—is old enough to have pubic hair, she's old enough to have sex with.

I've always disliked comparing sex to baseball, in part due to the sexist and heterosexist assumptions it makes. It sets up the idea that sex is a game and that there are opposing teams. The model relies on outdated gender stereotypes like boys are supposed to try to take the activity further and girls are gatekeepers who defend their turf. It turns sex into a competition. We're not playing on the same team; we're playing against each other—so someone wins, and someone loses. Another way to look at sexist gender roles in this model is to see boys as the players and the girls as the field upon which the game is played. For many young women in my class, the shock of this realization leaves them stunned, then sad, then angry.

It's also assumed that you play baseball in baseball season and when there's a game on the schedule. The timing isn't really up to you. So if it's prom night or if a teen's parents aren't home or someone's drinking at a party, the assumption is: Hey, it's batter up! If you're serious about playing baseball, you don't turn down the chance to get in the game. You don't sit on the bench just because you're tired or not in the mood to play. The expectation is that when you're called to bat, you'll be there.

And when we show up to play baseball, there's no need to discuss the rules or how you might want to play the game. Everybody is supposed to know how baseball works; you simply take your position and start playing. Rounding the bases is just what you do when you're dating. Some might argue that, when it comes to hooking up, "sliding into home" is what it's all about. Can you imagine a baseball player choosing to stay at second base when home plate is an option—even if they might like second base a whole lot better? Just like baseball, the assumption in sex is that everyone has the same priority: scoring. You move through first, second, and third base, not stopping until you slide home. There is an established order in which each activity happens. The baseball model also leaves no room for asexual or aromantic folks. It assumes that everyone wants to be involved in the game, and we know that's not true.

In this model, the decision to become sexually active is influenced more by external factors (this is how the game is played) than by internal factors (I'm ready, I'm committed to my sweetheart, and so on). It's not a decision being made by our kids for themselves. Often they're doing it because they're following what they *think* is the "right" model—the only model many kids have for sexual activity.

They think that rounding the bases is the only way to enjoy their sweetheart intimately. Many actually feel pressured into having intercourse simply because it's the "next" logical step. If

they don't want to have sex, the relationship isn't moving forward or growing the way they've been told it should, or they don't
really love their partner. I remember one student of mine who
came to me because she was terrified of telling her boyfriend she
wasn't ready to have sex. "He's going to think I'm a baby," she told
me. The decision not to have intercourse made her feel immature
in her circle of peers, which was ironic, of course, because her
thoughtful and informed decision actually made her one of the
more mature seniors in my class.

Sex as baseball isn't just sexist. It's heterosexist. It's competitive.
It's goal-directed, and it's unlikely to result in the development
of healthy sexuality in young people. It's also just plain negative.
After a game, there is the expectation of heading into the locker
room and rehashing the highlights—who performed well, where
the scorecard stands, who stole a base. Lots of kids don't like to
think about sex as a game. There's nothing in the baseball model
about consent or pleasure or intimacy or love. Nonetheless, most
kids feel they should be following it. I think part of the reason
this model has endured for so long is that it's clear-cut. When
you're in middle school and just trying to understand what various
sexual behaviors look like, it's helpful to have a straightforward,
chronologically ordered model to illustrate how it all works. Plus,
the baseball model offers an easily shared way of communicating
about a private subject. It feels less risky to chat casually with
friends about sexual activity if you can refer to intimate sex acts
as first, second, and third.

So what would it take for us to stop seeing sexual activity as a
challenge or a conquest?

A new model.

So I've cooked one up. It avoids the pitfalls inherent in the baseball model, and it's something I've talked about in packed roomfuls of parents, to youth-service providers at conferences, and even in a TED Talk. So here it is: instead of baseball, let's talk for a minute about pizza.

Did you smile when you read that? Did your mind conjure up a picture of your favorite pizza place, or a memory of eating really good pizza? That's the first good thing about my pizza model. Pizza is something that is widely and easily understood and something that most of us, including our kids, associate with a positive experience. The same can't be said for baseball. There are certainly fans of baseball who love it and immediately have positive associations with it, but I'll bet more people have a positive association with pizza.

To start, think about when you have pizza. Unlike baseball, whose schedule and rules are dictated from the outside, you have pizza when *you* want pizza. You eat it because you're in the mood for it. It starts with an internal sense, an internal desire, or a need. "Huh, I could go for some pizza!" The decision to act on the impulse rests with you—you are in control. I can recognize that I'm hungry but know that it's not a great time to eat. That ability to make a deliberate decision about our desire is a huge factor in developing healthy sexuality.

Another positive change in the pizza model is that when we get together with someone for pizza, we're not competing. We're looking for a shared experience that's satisfying for both of us. And even better, when you do decide to order a pizza with someone, what's the first thing you do? You talk about it. You talk about what you want; you talk about what they want; you may even negotiate.

"How do you feel about pepperoni?"

"Not really into it. I'm kind of a mushroom guy myself."

"Well, maybe we can go half and half?"

Even if you've had pizza with someone for a very long time, don't you still say things like, "Should we get the usual . . . or maybe something a little more adventurous?"

In other words, when you talk about sharing a pizza, you talk about desires and choices. You talk about the things that you both want, and you work together to make the best decision for both parties. Pizza puts you and your sweetheart on an equal footing. You're suddenly asking, "What's our pleasure?" What will taste good to both of us, and why? There are a million different kinds of pizza, a million different toppings, a million different ways to eat pizza. And none of them are wrong. They're different, and in this case different is good, because that's going to increase the chance that both people will have a satisfying experience.

And with pizza, there is no winner or loser—there is no competition. Shouldn't that be the model we use for sexual activity? Instead of rounding the bases, what if you asked: "Are we satisfied? Did we eat enough—did it taste good?" What makes us feel satisfied might be different amounts at different times. It might be different depending on whom we're sharing pizza with. But the key is that *we* get to decide when we feel satisfied. If we're still hungry, we might have some more. If we overindulge, we're likely to feel lousy. We have the power to make the decision that's best for us. Those decisions are also based in consent, something lacking in the baseball model. Nobody should force you to have pizza if you don't want it, and while sharing pizza, people can decide they've had enough, and that decision needs to be respected.

A lot of sexuality education in classrooms today is influenced by the baseball model. It's about forbidding kids from running the bases or, in more liberal programs, preparing students with contraceptives to protect against what is assumed to be the inevitability of intercourse. Either way, the baseball model supports the stereotype of boy as aggressor and girl as defender, and it's arming students with an unhealthy view of what it means to be sexually active. But if we could create sexuality education that was more like pizza, as I try to do in my class, we could create lessons that invite people to think about their own desires, to make deliberate decisions about what they want, to talk about their choices with their partners, and to ultimately look for not some external outcome, but for what feels satisfying.

In baseball, the coach, players, and umpire often yell out commands or judgments. "Stick close to the bag!" "Keep your eye on the ball!" "Strike three!" My pizza model is about asking questions. "What do you like on your pizza?" "How many slices do you want?" "Do you want to have pizza again tomorrow?" Learning about one's sexuality should be about assessing desires and asking and answering questions. That's what I hope you'll encourage your children to do as you read this book: ask and answer questions. I hope you'll encourage your kids to use pizza as their model for sexual activity: it's something to be enjoyed and explored and, ultimately, savored.

Normalizing the Sex Talks

During our lessons on sexual activity, I divide my students into four groups and give each group a different question to answer. The questions are: Why would boys your age have genital sexual activity (oral, vaginal, or anal)? Why would boys your age not have genital sexual activity (oral, vaginal, or anal)? Why would girls your age have genital sexual activity (oral, vaginal, or anal)? and Why would girls your age not have genital sexual activity (oral, vaginal, or anal)? As with all activities, I make it clear that answers should be inclusive of all sexual orientations. I also make clear to the students that this activity uses a binary conception of gender. Not all of my students identify their gender according to this binary. The activity doesn't presume that. I've tried adding questions about how people who identify as genderqueer, nonbinary, or agender would respond to the questions, but the majority of students don't know how to answer those questions. My goal here is to be able to talk about how we come to sexual activity with different assumptions and rationales. We can't assume that our partner thinks the same way about a sexual experience as we do, or prioritizes the same things about it. Often in the processing of the activity we talk about how folks with different gender identities and sexual orientations can have different ways of looking at sexual activity. So, even though the activity begins with a binary gender assumption, it doesn't end there.

The reasons might be different for same-gender and different-gender couples, or they might not be. The students huddle into their groups talking excitedly. I ask them first just to generate a list of as many answers to the question as they can. Don't judge them, just brainstorm away. After they've generated a long list, I ask them to select from their list what they believe are the top five answers to the question. The noise level in the room increases as they work to come to consensus to present to the class. I've found my students' answers throughout the years to be surprisingly similar. Remember as you read them, though, that these are just the responses I've gathered from my class. You might want to think about what your child and their friends' answers to the questions would be.

The top five reasons why boys would have genital sexual activity:

1. Because it feels good
2. Because you really like or love your sweetheart
3. To increase your reputation
4. Because you get caught up in the heat of the moment
5. Because societal expectations make you feel like you have to

The top five reasons why girls would have genital sexual activity are different:

1. Because she was asked to
2. Because she wants to keep a relationship going
3. Because she feels peer pressure from her friends or boyfriend
4. Because they're in love
5. Because they want to experiment or try new things

The top five reasons why boys wouldn't have genital sexual activity are:

1. They are insecure about their body or about their penis size
2. Religious beliefs
3. Questioning their sexual orientation (maybe they're gay and not yet out)
4. Fear of getting a girl pregnant
5. Insecure about their knowledge or ability to have sex

The top five reasons why girls wouldn't have genital sexual activity are:

1. Fear of pregnancy or STDs
2. Religious beliefs
3. Fear of getting a bad reputation
4. Haven't met the right partner yet
5. Fear that it will hurt

There are a lot of interesting assumptions in my students' answers. If boys are presented a chance to have genital sexual activity, there's no reason *not* to do it. It's rare to find a guy who says he's not ready for sex. Many heterosexual girls assume that the first time having intercourse is never pleasurable because "it's supposed to hurt." (By the way, many heterosexual boys also think that it's going to hurt for girls the first time, but they don't think about ways to avoid that either.) I frequently remind students that when sex is something both partners want, instead of something one or both feel pressured into doing, it's a much better experience, no matter what the sexual activity is. Having a conversation about why you're both into it can make it more pleasurable for everyone involved. Being fearful or overly anxious can make it less pleasurable. Notice also the heterosexist assumption that if a boy isn't having genital sexual activity, it might be because he's gay. I have to address that so we can make sure we're thinking about the full spectrum of diversity and including everyone in our ideas.

Now here's an interesting assumption that you may have about your teenager's sexuality: they're not supposed to feel pleasure. It can be scary to deviate from the baseball model for many parents, because otherwise they have to face the fact that their child may undress and seek sexual pleasure with another person. Remember when I mentioned in previous chapters that sex needs to be presented as a necessary and normal part of life? That means acknowledging that our children are sexual beings, that other people will be attracted to them, and that they will have feelings of attraction toward others. I know the thought of your child having sex may make you skittish. But don't even go that far. Let's begin by thinking about all of the other things that kids tend to do first: hold hands, make out, slow-dance. They're OK, right? Let's start there. Now jump ahead to when your child is in his or her twenties. Many parents tell me that they want their kids to fall in love, get married, and have children of their own someday. But someday doesn't just happen. There's a journey to get there, and it starts today. So how do we help young people take those first steps today? We talk to them about it. How do you do *that*? Here are a few ideas:

1. Don't talk about sex—yet. This may seem counterintuitive, but there are so many conversations you can have about sex without actually talking about naked bodies or intercourse. Remember, you're the person building the framework for their ideas about healthy sexuality. Talk about communication styles. Talk about love. Talk about news stories that relate to views on gender or sexual orientation. Remember, our sexuality is more than our genitals and what we do with them. To be able to get to those conversations, start with something broader, especially something that can give you an "in" to more direct conversations about sexual activity. The key is to start talking about *something* in a deliberate way.

2. Plan the talks, not the "Talk." Parents often think they have to sit down and have a formal talk about sex with their kids. Not so. As I discussed in the last chapter, those talks often backfire and can produce huge anxiety for everyone involved. Instead, think about having a conversation with your kids not in one long session, but in lots of small snippets. "Isn't it nice that Gloria on *Modern Family* lets her son, Manny, express his feminine side as well as his masculine side?" "Don't you think this ad of the woman in a bikini is ridiculous? Isn't it crazy how people fall in love on TV in ten minutes?" These kinds of ongoing interactions really give kids insight into their parents' values around sexuality without feeling as though they're being lectured. Also, your kids feel more connected to you when they realize that their parents think about some of the same things that *they* talk about with their friends. Just as you might have a hard time thinking about your child as a sexual being, believe me, your teenager has *no* interest in thinking about you as a sexual being either! But these kinds of casual remarks help them to see that you are, and you'll get a spark of recognition.

3. Try and try again. Many kids shut down their parents when they start to talk about sex, and eventually they just stop trying. Don't. Your children want to hear what you have to say, even if they act as though they're being tortured. Think of it like fishing. You're going to cast a whole lot of lines, patiently, before you get a nibble. Cast into the waters without expecting a response. When it's time to have bigger conversations, you'll both be ready and comfortable. And when you incorporate sexuality into your day-to-day conversations, you're sending an important message—that sex is a normal part of our existence. You're providing a healthy model for your kids' thoughts about sex.

4. Broadcast your feelings. I remember when I was younger and was watching a TV show with my mother. There was a gay character on the show, and I felt an affinity toward him. As we watched, I wanted one of my parents to say something, anything, about this character because it would help me place him in the larger world. "He's funny." "He's disgusting." "Oh, that poor man." But they said nothing, and the silence sent a huge message. If you're watching TV with your kids and there's a scene where a same-gender couple is expressing affection toward each other, you might say out loud: "Isn't that sweet?" or "Gee, they really seem happy together." Or whatever fits your own value set. You're giving your child context in which to place two gay characters. The same is true if a couple is heterosexual. If a couple is about to have sex on screen, don't get up and fill your water glass or suddenly stop speaking. Instead, give your children some idea of how you feel about it. "That's kind of an intense reaction to bringing donuts home, isn't it?" "I wouldn't want to hop into bed with somebody I just met." "Isn't he married to someone else?"

5. It's never too soon to start talking and keep talking. I can't emphasize enough how important it is to begin talking to your children about sexuality at a young age. And no age is too young. When preschool children play with their genitals, how you respond matters. When your third-grade daughter is called "flat," what you say can frame the way she thinks about her body and her sexuality. When your kids are looking at toy catalogs that divide the world strictly into boys' and girls' sections, will you affirm or challenge that notion? These are all conversations about sexuality, and it's important to take advantage of these moments so that your kids feel comfortable talking to you about sexuality as they grow older.

Infants, toddlers, and young children are naturally curious about their bodies and about the differences between theirs and others' bodies. Conversations with young children about sexuality and bodies can begin the moment they notice their genitals. In these early years, it's important to be upfront and open about what their body parts are and what they do. The most important things to remember when talking with young children are to take your cue from them, be sure you know what they're asking, and answer the question in as matter-of-fact a way as you can. Remember, when little ones don't know how to react to a situation, they look to you for clues. If you're upset, they're upset. If you seem scared, they'll feel fear. The more relaxed and comfortable you are, the more normal and healthy sexuality will seem to them. So for example, if it's your practice during bath time to name body parts as you wash them, don't make the genitals any different. "Now I'm washing your arm and your hand and your fingers. Now I'm washing your chest. Now I'm washing your vulva."

Let's look at a more extreme example—when you are the focus of sexuality. Let's say your seven-year-old walks into the bathroom while you're changing a tampon. What do you do? Again, take your cue from the child, who may think you're hurt. Many children would naturally associate blood with injury. You might just need to reassure them that Mommy's fine. If the child asks what the tampon is, say it's a tampon and it's something grown-up women use sometimes to help them stay clean and healthy. You can add that it's not anything little children need to use. You don't have to go into a detailed description of the menstrual cycle— your child isn't asking you for that information.

Young children will explore their bodies naturally. It feels good to touch themselves, and it's normal. It's your job to help them understand when it's appropriate to touch themselves (at home, in their bedroom, in the bath) and when it's not. If you're at the library and your daughter puts her hand down her pants, take her aside and explain why it's something reserved for home. "Honey, we only touch our vulva in private places like at home or in the bathroom. The library isn't a private place." If a child is too young to understand the difference between private and public, then they're too young to understand why you're trying to make them stop doing something they find soothing and pleasurable. In that case you can try substituting something else that's soothing and pleasurable. Treating bodies as shameful or secretive has negative effects on kids as they get older.

Many kids in elementary school will begin to wonder where babies come from. Obviously, all parents handle this question differently, but I suggest being open from the start. Rather than storks or doctors and nurses, try a G-rated version of the truth: "Mommies and daddies can bring their bodies together in a very special way to make a baby. It's not something that people your age can do yet, but when you're grown up you'll be able to do it." If you feel comfortable saying that making a baby entails Daddy's penis going into Mommy's vagina, that's a perfectly appropriate message.

6. Be sure you know what question your child is actually asking. I know a woman whose second-grader came into the kitchen and asked, "Mom, where did I come from?" Seizing the moment, Mom launched into a flurry of descriptions of birds, bees, seeds, and eggs. The youngster stared at her, puzzled, and said, "Oh, 'cause Amanda said she came from a hospital. Did I come from a hospital too?"

It turns out "Where did I come from?" was really the logistical question "Where was I born?" Likewise, the question "Can you get pregnant in a swimming pool?" might be a question about sex in public places, or about the spermicidal properties of chlorine, or a more general question about how pregnancy happens. Unless you take a moment to understand what question your child is really asking (which is tough to do if you become flustered), you might miss out on an opportunity to model healthy sexuality.

And once you understand the question, it's important to answer it directly—no beating around the bush or offering vaguenesses. Kids know how much information they want from us and are easily frustrated when they get too little or too much. A casual question deserves a casual answer; a specific question deserves a specific answer. Once you've answered the primary question, try to keep the dialogue going by asking open-ended questions. I guarantee, the question "Do you understand?" will elicit only a monosyllabic grunt. But saying, "I'd like to know what you think about that" or "Tell me if I answered your entire question" might have better results.

....

Question Box

Q: What would be considered "virginity" in the baseball model? How about the pizza model?

A: As with all questions about the term *virginity*, we should start by asking why the label *virgin* is important. What benefits and drawbacks come with that label? Are the benefits and drawbacks the same for people of all genders and sexual orientations? We might see sexism again here, as virginity is often seen as a desirable quality in women but not in men. Why is that? Is that fair?

In the baseball model, virginity usually has the definition of not having had vaginal sexual intercourse.

In the pizza model there is no standard definition of virginity. It would depend what the couple defines as "having sex." Remember, my definition for having sex is much broader—being involved with someone else's body for the purpose of giving and receiving sexual pleasure.

What does your definition of virginity tell you, and why does that answer matter?

Q: How many ninth-graders (by percentage) have pizza?

A: If by "pizza" you mean having vaginal intercourse, according to the Kaiser Family Foundation (a group that collects reliable data on sexual activity), about 6 percent of girls and 8 percent of boys have had intercourse by age fourteen. According to the Federal Interagency Forum on Child and Family Statistics 2021 report, the number of ninth-graders who have had sexual intercourse has actually declined. In the 1990s it was about 39 percent, but by 2021 that number has dropped to about 19 percent.* However, by the time they reach age nineteen, two out of ten teens have engaged in sexual intercourse. As you can see, what we said in class is true—the vast majority of students have not had vaginal intercourse by the end of their ninth-grade year.

....

* Federal Interagency Forum on Child and Family Statistics, *America's Children: Key National Indicators of Well Being, 2021*, U.S. Government Printing Office, https://www.childstats.gov/americaschildren21/index.asp.

Q: Do vulvas smell?

A: This is a very common question, but let's start by fixing the language. Many times this question is worded as "Do vaginas smell?" That may be what you're asking.

There is a myth out there that women's vaginas and vulvas may have an unpleasant smell. It is true that a vagina is home to a whole host of bacteria and other organisms, but these are supposed to be there—they're what make a vagina healthy! A healthy vagina or vulva will not have an unpleasant smell at all, but it will have a natural scent—just like all living things.

Here are a few other things to consider:

First, all human bodies smell, but not in a bad way! Our bodies are constantly secreting chemicals that give off odors. This is perfectly natural and normal; we're not sterile creatures! Places on our body that have hair are especially good at capturing our natural scent—that's one of the reasons we have hair where we do. Although humans do not have a very sensitive sense of smell, we do respond to those chemical signals that other people's bodies give off.

Second, all our natural scents are different. We will be more attracted to some than to others.

Third, the scent we give off can be a sign of how healthy or unhealthy we are. People who have a poor diet high in fat, people who smoke, people who abuse alcohol or drugs, or people who otherwise don't take good care of their bodies may have a scent to their skin and body fluids that is harsher, more acidic, and more bitter. People who have a healthy, balanced diet, who get regular exercise, and who don't smoke, drink, or take drugs will have a scent to their skin and body fluids that will range from mild to even somewhat sweet. So what you put into your body will be revealed one way or another.

Q: Why are hickeys pleasurable?

A: I'm not sure from your question what kind of pleasure you're talking about here, so I'll answer as broadly as I can. Starting with what exactly a hickey is.

A hickey is basically a bruise that is made by prolonged sucking or biting of a part of another person's body. Hickeys usually are found on the neck, but can be on any part of the body. And do you know what a bruise is? It results from breaking blood vessels on or near the surface of the skin. It's actually a minor injury. Hickeys are usually not harmful, but they can take several days to heal as the blood vessels that were broken mend themselves and the blood that's leaked out of them drains away. (Doesn't sound quite so sexy now, does it?)

Hickeys may be deliberately given or they may result from intense, passionate sexual activity in which people don't realize what they're doing.

In terms of the pleasure associated with them, getting a hickey may feel pleasurable because they usually occur on sensitive areas of the body that feel good when they're kissed or even nibbled a bit. The neck is a part of the body that is particularly sensitive to stimulation, and we often interpret that stimulation as sexual—especially when it occurs in a sexual situation. Giving someone a hickey may be pleasurable because our lips are also very sensitive, and when they touch sensitive skin, they are stimulated as well. So the good feeling can go both ways.

Despite the good feelings that may come from giving or getting a hickey, it also must be said that a hickey is usually given as a way of "marking" a person as yours. It's a way of saying, "You belong to me," which is pretty oppressive when you think about it. It can be used as a way of showing power over one's partner (Look what I can do) or showing an unequal level of power in the relationship (I'm in charge). When hickeys are used in this way, I think they're pretty awful.

Q: Is it normal to just randomly get turned on throughout the day multiple times a day? P.S., I'm a girl, not a guy.

A: Not only is this normal, it's perfectly healthy. Every person, guy or girl, has a personal threshold of sexual arousal. Some people get turned on pretty easily, so it's natural for them to feel that way many times in a day. Other people get turned on less frequently. Also remember that our regular level of arousal is influenced by a host of factors, including our physical and mental state. We can all go through periods when we're more or less turned on than what's usual for us.

The other thing to remember is that there are a variety of ways to deal with being turned on. Some people masturbate. Some people fantasize. Some people try to think about something unsexy to get their mind off of sex. We all need a variety of strategies for dealing with desire, especially in situations where it's not welcome.

....

CHAPTER 4

Love and Relationships: Becoming Your Authentic Self

Before class one day, I observed a small group of girls discuss the relationship status of one of their friends.

"Are they together?" asked someone.

"No."

"So they're just hooking up?"

"No. They have a thing."

"Oh."

Amazingly, that seemed to clarify the situation for the girls, and they moved on to other topics. I, however, was lost.

"Wait," I interrupted. "They have a *thing*? What thing?" Usually I'm pretty good at decoding teenage idioms. I am, after all, an English teacher in addition to a sexuality educator. But I had no idea what they were talking about.

The girls looked at me with a kind of pity they reserve for a naive child or a hopelessly out-of-touch old person.

"Mr. V, you don't know what a thing is?"

Desperately trying to sound cool, smart, and smooth, the best I could say was, "Well, a thing can be a lot of things, can't it?"

They, of course, saw right through me.

"No, we're not talking about things in general. They have *a thing*."

"Is a thing a relationship?" I asked, grasping at straws.

They sighed and gave me that look of pity again.

"No, a thing is when you're not in a relationship but you're more than just hooking up with someone."

"Oh, so they're dating," I said with some sense of assurance. I finally thought I understood.

"Mr. Veeeeee," the girls giggled. "Nobody *dates* anymore."

"Well, it's a good thing we're headed into the love and relationship unit," I said. "Clearly, I have a lot to learn."

What Kind of Relationship Is This?

When we begin the relationship unit in my class, the students assume we're going to start with romantic and sexual relationships. We're not. Those are the relationships they're most hungry to understand, but we need a much wider context in which to place those relationships before we can begin to talk about them. Romantic and sexual relationships don't exist in a vacuum. They're influenced by all of the other kinds of relationships in our lives. We're more than just sweethearts; we're mothers and fathers, sisters and brothers. We're friends, neighbors, bosses, and students. When we examine these nonsexual and nonromantic relationships first, we can see how they influence and are connected to the romantic and sexual ones. It's also important to start with nonsexual and nonromantic relationships because more and more kids are identifying as asexual or aromantic (which they abbreviate as "ace" or "aro"). Not every person wants or needs to be in a romantic or sexual relationship, and that's fine.

So I start this unit by asking students to think about the many different types of relationships they have in their lives, what they expect out of each one, and why. Relationships, especially nonromantic, nonsexual ones, are something you can take for granted when you're seventeen: Your parents are just *there*. Your high school friends are your world, and you think they always will be. But when you're having your first serious sexual and/or romantic relationship, you're dealing with lessons about love, commitment, responsibility, jealousy, and manipulation, and at the end of it, how to cope with the inevitable broken heart. You're learning a new relationship role and discovering what it feels like to be on the other end of someone else's relationship role. The only context we have for helping us understand and process all of those new roles and feelings is the relationships we already have in our lives. That's the starting point.

But there's another problem with beginning a discussion of relationships with the romantic and sexual ones: within the romantic and sexual category there are many varieties of relationships—friendship, hooking up, friends with benefits, a *relationship*, even a "thing." And while my students are able to make a list of all of these different terms, they're not always good at distinguishing the differences among them. For example, they define a hookup as someone you are sexual with once or twice, with no emotional or romantic engagement. A friend with benefits, though, is a friend with whom you do have emotional engagement, but whom you also hook up with on a recurring basis—with no "relationship" strings attached. If that's confusing to you, imagine what it's like for them. They're not so good at differentiating each type of relationship, and they have an even harder time figuring out how to tell when a relationship is changing from one thing into another. Talking about the pros and cons of each kind of relationship objectively is also tough for them. That's why we start at square one.

A psychologist named Robert Sternberg offers a helpful theory about love that I like to use to talk to my students about relationships. He says that love has three components: intimacy, passion, and commitment—I think that's a handy rubric for talking about all kinds of relationships.* Sternberg defines intimacy as the emotional aspect of a relationship. I call it the heart-to-heart connection. It's the part of you that wants to be close to the other person and feel connected to them. Passion (what I call the body-to-body connection) is the desire for sexual expression and pleasure with each other. The last aspect is commitment. That's the intellectual aspect of a relationship. I call it the mind-to-mind connection. There's short-term commitment, when you're deciding whether or not to take one more step in the relationship, and long-term commitment, when you dig in for the long haul, which, for a teenager, may be a year or even six months. This is a good gauge

---

* R. J. Sternberg, "A Triangular Theory of Love," *Psychological Review* 93, no. 2 (1986): 119–35.

for kids to begin thinking about different relationships, because almost every relationship we have incorporates one or more of these aspects.

So in my class, we start off the relationship unit by talking about the lowest level of relationship, an *acquaintance*. The acquaintance relationship doesn't typically embody any of Sternberg's categories. These are people who don't turn you on (and if they do, you're unlikely to do anything about it). You have no desire for an intimate connection with them, and you're not actively doing anything to keep the relationship going. It's amazing how many people in our lives fit into this category. For my students, acquaintances can range from a kid they see on the school bus each morning or afternoon to the many adults who cross their paths during a day (like some teachers). They're the people who take their orders in restaurants and can even be the people they watch on TikTok or whom they're connected to via social media.

The next level of relationship we talk about is a *nonromantic friend*, or friend *without* benefits. These people would rate low on passion; we're not usually turned on by our friends, but there's often high intimacy in a friendship. With friends, we do quite a bit of emotional sharing back and forth. Our commitment level with friends can vary; some of our friends are there for the rest of our lives, but some, like many of our high school friendships, are shorter-term connections.

Then there's *hooking up*. My students would say that hooking up is high on the passion scale but low on intimacy and commitment, for it's about the physicality of the moment, not what happens before or after. Adults might refer to this kind of a relationship as a one-night stand. It means you're not interested in knowing too much about each other—you just want the body-to-body connection, and you want it now.

When you're *seeing somebody* or *hanging out with somebody* or *having a* thing *with somebody*, as my students would call it, the language gets fuzzy. It's high passion with rising intimacy, but there's also short-term commitment. You're typically attracted to the person and want it to be more than "just a hookup," yet you're not in a long-term relationship.

Being in a sweetheart relationship checks all the boxes: it's high on passion, high on intimacy, and has long- or short-term commitment—what's essential is that there's emotional and physical commitment to each other. My students can easily *say* what a relationship is, but they haven't always given a lot of thought to what it actually *means* to be in a relationship.

Now, of course, these are fairly arbitrary categories. The reality of our relationships is more fluid. My students push back against absolutes. They're quick to note that the edges of all these categories can meld into each other, and that's true. Acquaintances can become friends; friends can become sweethearts; sweethearts can become acquaintances. It's always best, my wise young pupils remind me, to think of this more like a continuum with an infinite variety of combinations. They're smart cookies, my kids. They're also terrified of feeling boxed in and will squirm mightily to twist themselves out of having to define a relationship they're in. Hence their quandary about *friends with benefits*.

My students are always tripped up when they try to put *friends with benefits* into Sternberg's categories. As a parent, you should know that *friends with benefits* is pretty common among young people, though that doesn't mean it's a model that actually works for them. Just to be clear, *friends with benefits* means you're friends who can be sexual together without ever moving into a *thing* or a "real relationship." My students know when they're hooking up with somebody, and they know when they're in a relationship, but what they can't describe is how one turns into the other, the moment when a relationship starts. Here's why it's tough for them to deconstruct: when you're in a friends-with-benefits relationship, the passion is there, and the emotional intimacy is there, but they quickly discover that romantic intimacy is very different from friendship intimacy.

"Your lover can be your friend, but can your friend be your lover?" I'll ask them. I often push teenagers to share why many of them rely on the friends-with-benefits model of relationships. To me, it's a cop-out. If I really push them to explain why their romantic relationships often default to it, many will admit as much. "You get all of the good stuff that a relationship has, but you don't have to do the hard work," a student once told me.

There are drawbacks and benefits to all of the relationships we have. When talking about relationships (and we talk about this in some detail in class), I don't judge the hookup versus the long-term sweetheart. A healthy person will have many of these types of relationships over the course a lifetime. There's no one "right" relationship for everyone, no one goal to which we all should aspire. However, I do think it's important to have some idea of what you might want your future to look like, and use that as a way of informing the decisions you make and assessing where you want to be when it comes to your sexual and romantic relationships.

"When you think about the future, you know, when you're (God forbid) as old as me," I'll ask my students, "how many of you picture yourself working on your third divorce?"

Nobody raises a hand.

"How many of you want to live alone with a lot of cats?"

One or two kids raise their hands. "A fine goal, if that's what you want," I say. "But what *do* you want for your future?"

They'll blurt a few variations on the same answer: they want a relationship that's fun and sexy, full of support and pleasure, one that's stable and loving and that they can depend on.

"Keeping that long-term goal in mind, I want you to think about the path from here to where you want to end up. If you've mastered the hookup, that brings a certain set of skills, but does it bring you the skills to get to your relationship goal?"

"Part of the way there," a boy with a goatee says.

"Sure," I say. "But if you want to be a good basketball player, why are you practicing on your skateboard all of the time? At the end of the day, you'll simply be a good skateboarder who wishes he could play basketball."

I let that sink in. Then continue: "All of the relationships we have in life offer us opportunities to practice, to learn from our mistakes, and to grow. Relationships, whether friendships or sweethearts, don't just happen; they require work. The only way we can become more knowledgeable about relationships—and thereby our role in them—is by being in relationships, and by being our authentic selves in those relationships."

"Great!" a sly guy interrupts. "You just said we have to practice hookups, so I'm gonna practice and practice and practice and tell my mom you said it was OK."

I turn to one of the more mature members of the class and ask, "Is that what I said?"

"Nope," he confirms with a shake of his head.

"Just to be clear," I say with deliberateness, "if you're looking to me to tell you what kind of relationship you can or should be in, then I don't think you're ready for any kind of sexual relationship. I'm not saying everyone needs to have a hookup while they're in high school. Only you can decide what kind or level of relationship you're ready for. Part of what this class is all about is giving you a framework to figure that out. Some people may decide they never want to have a hookup at any point in their lives, but especially in high school."

That statement brings an interesting mix of responses. Some kids snort in derision; others visibly relax, relieved of one particular burden in the midst of a life that already seems too complicated.

Building Healthy Relationships: What Is Your Bottom Line?

As adults, we've likely fallen in and out of love, survived heartbreak, fallen into bed with somebody we knew wasn't right for us. All of these interactions helped shape us into who we are today. While many teenagers think they know everything about, well, everything, an important part of coming of age is understanding what you want out of relationships (and life, for that matter) and, more important, what you *don't* want out of relationships (and life). So begin our conversations about deal breakers and deal makers.

When you live in a hypersexualized culture like ours, there's pressure to be paired off to feel accepted by peers and society at large, even if that pairing is a friends-with-benefits situation. Our discussion about deal makers and deal breakers is really a conversation about what teens are willing to accept in a relationship and what they're not and how those limits inform their decisions about their sexuality. For example, some kids know even as young as sixteen that they'll never be in a long-term relationship with someone who is not of their religion. I've had many of my Jewish students tell me they'd never marry someone who doesn't share their faith tradition. That's a real deal breaker.

Other kids won't know how to answer me when I ask if they have any deal breakers when it comes to relationships. A few will always wonder aloud if they have any deal breakers at all. I challenge them to think harder—nearly all of us have something that would end a relationship, or seal it. Maybe it's your sweetie's age. Are you willing to date someone a decade older? What about younger? If your partner physically pushed you during a fight, would that be the end of the relationship for you? What if your partner made fun of your little sister? It's also important for kids to know that some deal makers and deal breakers can change as we grow. Others will remain set in stone no matter what our age. Thinking about our individual deal makers and deal breakers in relationships is an evolving process. We continually need to call them to mind, evaluate them, and make adjustments when necessary.

Parents often have quite a few bottom-line ideas when it comes to healthy relationships, and rightly so. Parents may not like their child's older beau, or they may dislike the negative attitude of their new sweetheart. But your kids expect you to set limits—it's essential in helping them learn what's right and what's not. This is true for their relationships, as well. In the best case, you can have a conversation with your child about your concerns and try to come to a mutually agreeable solution, but as a parent, you can also say to your child: "I don't like this person you're hanging out with. I don't want you to see them." It's also OK to seek out information about someone your child is spending a lot of time with. For example, ask the other parents on the sidelines of your child's next sporting event what they've heard about a kid you're worried about, or ask an older sibling about a younger child's friends. Depending on the rules you've established with your child about online privacy, it might also be appropriate to look at their social media or the texts on their phone.

Still, a parent walks a fine line when expressing an opinion about a child's relationships. Say the wrong thing, and your child may simply get angry and push you away. It's best to help the child do some critical analysis so they comes up with the conclusion on their own. For example: If your tenth-grade daughter suddenly grows close to a mean girl, it's OK to say you don't like how her friend treats people. Then find more subtle ways to bring it up in conversation. If you once had a mean girl treat you badly, share the story. Kids respond incredibly well to stories about how their parents handled similar situations.

It's much better to have a conversation about healthy relationships—what makes good relationships good—than a talk about what's wrong with your son or daughter's friend. I spend a few weeks teaching kids what it means to be in a healthy relationship, so they have some basis for recognizing the types of relationships they find themselves in and what the possible pros and cons are of any relationship. One of the problems that I see today is that kids don't have a real sense of what a healthy relationship should look like, how to get into one, and how to get out of an unhealthy one. That's partially because they have so few role models. Many have parents who have split, their peers are equally clueless, and the relationships they see portrayed in the movies or "reality" TV aren't exactly real.

When I define what I mean by a "healthy relationship" with my class, the first thing I say is that the relationship *must* have equitable levels of power. I don't say equal, because I don't think they'll ever be exactly equal when it comes to factors like money, age, and sexual experience. In a high schooler's world, power often depends on who has a license, how late someone's curfew is, whose parents let their child drink in the basement with friends. For a classic example of a power imbalance, take the senior dating a ninth-grader. This is a problematic relationship for many reasons, but mostly because that relationship will never be close to equal in power. Ninth-graders can't drive, twelfth-graders can. The older kids know their way around the school better, they have more friends, and often more sexual experience. It's nearly impossible for a twelfth-grader *not* to take advantage of a ninth-grader in the same way that it's hard for a ninth-grader not to give in to a twelfth-grader. The relationship is unequal. When I challenge kids to think about why this relationship is not a healthy one, they often push back.

"What if it's a really mature ninth-grader and an immature twelfth-grader?" they'll ask.

"What if the younger person has more social power than the older one?"

"What if the ninth-grader is the one with more sexual experience?"

I find when arguing with teenagers, it's helpful to use sources of information they respect, and that often means the Internet. When they push back about older-younger relationships, I ask them, "In your time surfing the Web, haven't you come across that formula that tells you the age of the youngest person a person should date?" They nod their heads, and someone always yells out, "Half your age plus seven!"

I am uncertain of the origin of this "rule," but it's actually a helpful guideline for kids in high school. If you're fourteen, then you should be dating someone who is fourteen. If you're eighteen, you shouldn't be dating someone under sixteen—and only a handful of ninth-graders are sixteen. Of course there's always someone who will note that most seniors are seventeen, and according to the formula, they can date someone who's fifteen and a half. My response is simple.

"You always round up."

Another critical component of a healthy relationship, I tell them, is maintaining your individuality within the relationship. I try to stress to my students the difference between being two people in a relationship and being a relationship of two people. Don't see the difference? Look at what comes first in each sentence. "Two people in a relationship" is about two individuals coming together to create a third entity (the relationship) that exists in addition to themselves as individuals. In a "relationship of two people," each partner's individuality is subsumed into the greater relationship. There's a great example of this in the comic strip *Zits* by Jerry Scott and Jim Borgman. RichandAmy are described on the strip's website as "an inseparable couple unanimously considered as one organism." They're drawn in a perpetual embrace, together all the time, and can't make a move without the other person being involved. My shorthand for these couples is that they "share a lung" and can't breathe if they get too far away from each other.

In so many teenage relationships, there's an expectation that your sweetie comes first, above your friends, schoolwork, sports. I often tell my students: "You shouldn't be with your sweetheart 24-7." You may want to, but it's not a good idea. Each person is allowed to have friends and interests and time away from the other. I ask those students in relationships to take a challenge. For the next twenty-four hours, I'll tell them, I don't want you to text your sweetie more than once every two hours. Most can't do it. It's not just because they're a wired generation and default to text rather than talking (which we'll address later). It's because they haven't developed a sense of trust or security in their relationship. They need everything to be validated over and over again. Living that way causes an incredible amount of anxiety, and I don't think it's healthy. Also, that constant contact when directed toward a significant other can be a form of power. *Where are you? What are you doing? Who are you with? When will you be home?* In extreme cases, it can even morph into a form of bullying, harassment, or abuse. It's hard to say to a friend or sweetheart, "I have soccer after school, then I have to do my homework and go to bed. Talk to you tomorrow," and then to ignore the flurry of status updates and countertexts that will come their way in the minutes and hours later. This point isn't just about electronic communication, though. It's important for anyone to be able to express and pursue one's own needs, wants, and interests while in a relationship. When each partner claims personal power and individuality, the possibility of an abusive or enmeshed relationship is lessened. While it's hard at first for teens to understand that this healthy division doesn't make them any less committed to the relationship, learning to balance their own identity with their identity as half of a couple is an important skill for young people to develop.

Some kids will argue that they can carry on a romantic relationship largely through e-mails, status updates, and texts. I tell them that makes me uncomfortable. They tell me I'm old and out of touch. I believe if two people have the option of face-to-face meetings but choose an alternative way to be together, like texting or FaceTiming, it's fair to ask why. I challenge students to think about why they're choosing to text so much with a sweetheart. Is it because it's less awkward? Sometimes I think kids use the Internet as a crutch to avoid the work of relationships. If you want to be in a long-term romantic relationship, you have to figure out how to be in the same room together and talk to each other without the filter of a screen. You have to push through the awkward moments. When you're sixteen or seventeen, the worst thing in the world is feeling awkward—after all, you are terribly self-conscious most of the time, but at the deepest level, you simply want to be loved and accepted. But as I tell my students over and over again, "Real life is awkward!" and the only way to deal with awkwardness is to walk through it and come out the other side. They push back mightily against this idea, yet it does eventually sink in. On a visit back to the school during a college break, one of my former students told me that the most important lesson he took away from the class was that life was awkward and that was OK. He said it allowed him to be so much more authentic with friends and sweethearts; he didn't have to try to be perfect. He could just be himself and go from there.

Another component of a healthy relationship: being able to express both positive and negative feelings, comments, and opinions to your sweetheart. We disrespect teenagers sometimes by saying that they don't know what they want, but sometimes they do, and it's an important life skill to know that you can own those feelings. If a young person really does want to have sex with their sweetheart, they should be able to say so without being coy. Similarly, a young person who is fine with kissing and cuddling shouldn't feel the need to have sex with their sweetheart to feel good about the relationship. Even though a friend relationship is different from a romantic relationship, I remind kids that there should be the same level of comfort and honesty. "Would you think twice about telling a friend that you can't talk because you need to study? When your friend asks what movie you want to see, don't you tell them what you really want rather than what you think they want to hear? It should be the same with your sweetheart." My mentor in graduate school, Dr. Kenneth George, studied love. He said the best way to define romantic love was "best friend + sex." I amend and clarify that slightly for my students to "best friend qualities + sexual desire." I tell my students that their sweetheart doesn't have to be their best friend, but that their relationship should reflect the same qualities—honesty, ease, and joy.

One way that parents can inspire their kids to practice expressing themselves is by giving them choices and really encouraging them to say what they want as opposed to what parents want for them. *Do you want to go to church or stay home? We're going to your sister's soccer game—are you interested in joining us?* Whether it's allowing them to choose their own clothes or giving them a weekly allowance to manage, in these small ways, you're helping them build a strong sense of self and practice voicing their own wants and needs.

Reliable commitment patterns are the last quality of healthy relationships that I teach. "If I say I'm going to do something for a friend, and I don't, I'll be marked as unreliable," I'll tell my kids. It's important that people show up when they say they're going to show up, that they call when they say they're going to call. There's responsibility in relationships, whether it's a sweetheart relationship or a friendship. I want them to know that it's important for them to consider their own behaviors as much as they do those of their significant others. It's easy to forgive our sweethearts and make excuses for them when they don't live up to our expectations, but it's important to see the relationship with clear eyes and remind ourselves that we deserve reciprocity. If a sweetheart isn't treating us the way that we treat them or want to be treated, it's probably time to have a serious talk or reconsider the relationship.

For many of us, adults included, the beginning of a relationship is a magical period. We work hard to not see the flaws in each other and to reveal only our best traits. We groom ourselves meticulously. You give your sweetie all of your attention while ignoring those little quirks that otherwise might annoy you. But as time goes on, there's a point at which you have to give up that illusion of perfection. Here's the way I address this in class: "You can only hold in a fart for so long," I tell my students. They howl, yet they know exactly what I mean. There's only so long that you can snuggle with each other on the couch or play together in bed before somebody farts. You think, *Who are you? What is this person?* It's the moment when our authentic selves begin to come out, because there's only so long that any of us can hide behind this idea that we're perfect. Real and authentic people are imperfect. "If a relationship is going to last and become long-term," I tell my students, "you have to be willing to acknowledge and engage with the imperfect person." This is also a great moment to make a related point. Nobody in porn is ever awkward, right? Nobody ever leans on someone's hair or gets a cramp. It's just not reality.

Reassure your kids that they're not supposed to have it all figured out. They're not going to be relationship experts or navigate relationships perfectly the first few times out of the gate. That's not a realistic expectation to put on teens. All we can expect them to do is try to create healthy patterns of relationships. And we can tell them that it's OK to stand up for your bottom line. Sometimes the hardest part about being a kid is finding the strength to admit that you're different or that you don't want to do something that everybody else is doing. It's the push and pull of adolescence— you want to find out who you are, but deep down you hope that you're just like everybody else.

Many students sometimes find themselves in situations where they're asked to do something that doesn't feel OK, and I push them to trust their instincts. Many of them can acknowledge that deep down inside something doesn't feel right. "You're the best gauge for what's normal in your relationship," I tell my class. "You're the expert in your life. When you do something based upon your own values, that's powerful stuff." Many of my students nod appreciatively when they hear this. I remember one student saying, "Wow, I didn't know I could trust myself with this stuff."

"If you don't feel like you're being your authentic self, if something doesn't feel right about the relationship, whatever it is, then it's OK to name that thing and deal with it. What if your younger sibling was in the same situation—what advice would you give them?"

Surviving Their First Breakup

Several years ago there was a young man in my class who was experiencing his first broken heart. The girl he had been dating for over two years, his first "true love," had broken up with him. While she wasn't in our class, she was at our school, and he couldn't avoid running into her or seeing her on campus. He came to see me one day, and my heart ached to see him so sad and upset. On the verge of tears, he asked for advice on what to do, how to get over feeling so devastated. What I said to him seemed like common sense to me but was a revelation for him.

"I can see how sad you are about this," I said. "Are you letting yourself be sad? Have you cried about it?"

"No," he said. "My friends all tell me to cheer up and get over it. They say I shouldn't let her make me sad, that I should be strong. I try hard to smile and look like I'm OK."

I looked at him and said gently, "I think you should let yourself be sad. It's a really sad thing that's happened. It hurts so much because what you felt for her was real. If you didn't really care about her you would be able to just get on with things. But you did and still do care about her, don't you?"

He sniffled and nodded.

"So let it out. It's OK. It's honest and it's what you need to do." He crumpled onto his desk and sobbed. I patted his head, handed him tissues, and waited. After a good cry, he lifted his head.

"Nobody told me it was OK to be sad," he said through tears still streaming down his cheeks.

"What else can you be right now?" I asked. "Allowing yourself to be sad and to express it is the only way the sadness will end."

Although adults may not think that their kids are capable of forming "real" relationships, high school relationships are very real to your kids. To suggest anything else is disrespectful. They may not be at the same level of intimacy and depth as romantic relationships in our adult years, but to your kids, they're every bit as emotional and important. A six-month relationship may feel goofy to us. But to your kids, six months is an eternity.

"Can you be in love when you're sixteen?" your children may ask you. Of course you can. But I'm not sure it's the same kind of love you might share with someone when you're twenty-five. I often encourage parents to have a talk with their children about what it means to be in love at sixteen or seventeen, and how it's different from being in love when you're older. A breakup is a good time to talk about the lessons of love. Part of building a healthy sexuality is helping kids walk through these experiences in their early years, when there's less at stake and they have people around who can guide them. Another critical move you can make as a parent: acknowledge that there is a process that people go through when relationships end and give your kids permission to feel their feelings.

Albert Angelo, a longtime friend and fellow sexuality educator, offers a perspective on breakups that I find helpful when speaking to my students. He suggests that after a relationship ends, people go through emotional stages very similar to Elisabeth Kübler-Ross's model of the stages of grief. Thinking about it in this way makes clear what a powerful life event a breakup can be and why so many of us can still feel a tinge of pain years after a relationship has ended and we have moved on. When I offer students this perspective, it helps them feel that they're not crazy, that it's normal to feel the way they do, and that their emotions are legitimate. Another nice thing about using this model as a reference is that it speaks to both parties in the relationship—the one initiating the breakup and the one on the receiving end of it. When we're face-to-face with a young person who's hurting from a breakup, it can be very helpful to be familiar with this model. It gives us a framework for a conversation that will be helpful as well as comforting. It's also important for young people to know about this model so that they aren't blindsided by the feeling they experience when they have that inevitable first breakup.

8 Stages of Grief and Healing After a Breakup

1. Denial

Even though at some level one or both partners know the relationship is in trouble, it can be frightening to admit there's a problem. If the problems can be brought out into the open and addressed, the couple could try to work on the relationship. Sadly, this may not happen. In addition, one partner may actively hide feeling unhappy and wanting to leave the relationship in order to "not rock the boat" and/or to secretly plan an exit strategy. That deception may help the other partner stay in denial. But when the denial breaks, the pain begins.

2. Anger and Confusion

The person who will initiate the breakup may feel frustrated by the other. Just being around that person can be enough to make the initiator feel annoyed. Personality quirks and other qualities that were never a problem start to get on their nerves. The person who will be on the receiving end of the breakup may feel genuinely confused as to why their sweetheart suddenly seems so angry or upset all the time. When the breakup does occur, the partner on the receiving end may react in angry outbursts, such as "You can't do this to me!" "I won't let you go!" or even "I hate you!"

3. Bargaining: We Can Work It Out

This is when both people realize the relationship is in trouble and might be coming to an end. Even for the person who wants to break up, it's scary. Things look bad, but sometimes you might think you can fix it. When that doesn't happen, the person on the receiving end of the breakup may become obsessed with trying to mend the relationship and win back the other, resorting to bargaining: "Please don't leave until we graduate from high school" or "Can't we wait and decide whether to break up after the summer's over?" Couples may repair a relationship at this stage if both really want to do so. A relationship will continue when both partners believe the work of staying together is worth it. A relationship will end when at least one partner believes staying together is just too much work. It takes two to stay together but only one to break apart.

4. Acknowledgment and Grieving

This stage can begin only when a person admits the relationship is over—the denial has ended. It is in this stage that grief is felt most acutely and most deeply. As I told the brokenhearted young man who came to see me, "If you're feeling bad, it's because what you had was real. If it didn't matter, it wouldn't hurt so badly." I also reminded him, "When you're hurting, you're healing." While both parties experience some level of grief, the one who is left may experience more and deeper levels of it in the form of abandonment and rejection, and the sense of not being good enough to keep a sweetheart from leaving.

5. Evaluation: What Went Wrong?

Grief offers an opportunity to shine a light in the dark, painful space of the breakup and look at what went wrong. It's like an emotional autopsy. The person who initiated the breakup may begin to experience some feelings of regret, recognizing that there were good aspects to the relationship—it wasn't all terrible. And after some time apart, the initiator may come to miss their sweetheart. (Note: I'm happy when kids can get this far in the process. They're not always emotionally equipped to continue from here.)

For the person who was on the receiving end of the breakup, this stage often offers a time to reflect on what wasn't great about the relationship. Many of my students come to realize during their grief that their ex wasn't perfect, and that being out of the relationship may have some unexpected benefits. They may realize how their stress level has declined, or how they don't have to keep a tally of time spent with a sweetheart versus time spent with friends. They may even realize that they feel happy, something they may not have felt in a while, especially during the earliest stages of the breakup.

6. I'm Not the Same Person

In relationships, you can sometimes forget your own individual strengths and likes. Once the relationship ends, it's normal to try to reconnect with your old self. *I love to paint but I never had time to paint when I was with them. I like to cook at home but they always wanted to go out to dinner.* This is a stage that offers both parties the opportunity to grow and develop into their most authentic selves as they rediscover the interests and personality traits that make them who they are. However, this can be a tricky stage for teenagers to understand, as most teens are still forming their identities.

7. There's No Going Back

In this stage a person accepts that it was right that the relationship ended. Breaking up wasn't a mistake. We all know that this becomes easier as you get older, but in our early relationships, we don't always have the perspective or life experience to know that ending a relationship that wasn't working is the right thing to do. It's helpful to let your children know that life gets better and that happiness is in moving forward and opening their hearts again.

8. Peace

You can interact with or be around your ex and not feel bitter or angry or disgusted, as many teens initially do. When they reach this stage, it's important to communicate that they don't need to feel any ill will toward a former sweetheart. After all, they're going to be around each other a lot if they go to the same school, and when teens are angry about a breakup, they can be cruel to each other. Because many teens (and quite a few adults) will never get to this stage in the process, and because we live in an age where momentary rage can be crystallized forever on social media, when rumors can be circulated in seconds, it's especially important that we help young people quell the desire to lash out, hurt, or even bully their exes or their exes' friends. You don't have to be completely at peace with a breakup to know that deliberate cruelty will only make things worse. My students often ask me, "What are the signs that a relationship is going badly?" I tell them that one warning sign to look out for is a shift in the balance of power to a less equitable arrangement. When your sweetie seems to be more interested in criticizing you than in complimenting you, it's usually the beginning of the end. Teasing can also be a sign. Friends tease us in a loving way all the time, but sometimes with a sweetie, teasing becomes something that feels bad. It pushes the two of you apart. These are all behaviors that may escalate at the end of a relationship, but they don't need to continue after a relationship is over if both parties can achieve peace.

I often tell kids that relationships don't last forever, at least not when you're in high school. While I acknowledge to them that their relationships are important, I remind them that they don't have to go into them with the expectation that they'll be with these persons for the rest of their lives. When kids stop thinking that their ninth-grade sweeties will someday meet them at the altar, some of the pressure of young love lifts. And while I'm not advocating all sorts of experimentation at a young age, I do want my students to know that it's OK to try out different relationships and get to know different kinds of people. It's not until they've lived through a few breakups and makeups that they'll begin to learn what kind of relationship is best for them.

Question Box

Q: I want to have a relationship with someone, but I don't know how to talk to them or "put myself out there." Do you have any tips?

A: The first thing I'd say is, don't go into an interaction with the purpose of getting into a relationship. That puts a ton of pressure on everyone involved. Start by just trying to make a casual, honest connection with the person. Strike up a conversation about something you like and feel comfortable talking about. Ask them questions about themselves. The more "chill" you can be, the more natural the interaction will be, and the better the groundwork will be laid for something more to develop. Relationships that evolve are a lot less stressful and more successful than those we try to force into existence.

Sweetheart relationships should be based on honesty, so don't play games with people. Say what you feel and mean what you say. If you like someone, tell them. That may seem scary, but it's the best way to get an honest reaction in response.

Q: Is it unhealthy to *not* have a romantic relationship until after high school, or should you just jump into it and then see how it all goes?

A: It's perfectly healthy to go through high school without having a romantic relationship—or any kind of sexual relationship, for that matter. What would be unhealthy is forcing yourself to do it because of some idea that you "should." Some people just don't want or feel ready for a relationship while in high school. That's perfectly fine. I would say it's important to examine your values, stay open to all the possibilities, and see what happens. You may not be ready now, but there's a lot of high school left. You might feel differently in a year or so, and you might not. Either way is fine.

Q: I haven't had my first kiss yet. Is this a problem?

A: No problem at all! There's no "right" age to have a first kiss. It can happen at any age. If it hasn't happened for you yet, then it hasn't happened.

I imagine you might feel pressure to have that first kiss, but don't do it just for the sake of doing it (or just to get it over with). You deserve to have it with someone you really *want* to kiss. And when you find that person, be sure to let them know that you've selected them to share your first kiss—that's an honor! If they don't treat it like the amazing gift it is, then they don't deserve to be your first kiss.

I know there's someone out there who would feel really special to be part of your first kiss. That's who you deserve!

Q: Is it normal to be in love with someone and be very attracted to them but some weeks not feel nearly as attracted and as desperate to talk to them, etc.?

A: What you're describing is absolutely normal! Relationships with sweethearts don't exist in a vacuum; they are constantly being influenced and affected by things happening to us and around us. On any given day, our emotional state—whether we're tired or stressed or upset with a family member—can affect how attracted we feel to our sweethearts. If our sweetheart is feeling stressed or sick or grumpy, that can affect how much we feel attracted to them as well. Being in a relationship doesn't mean that we're always attracted to our sweetheart the same amount all the time. We're all human; we don't stay in any emotional state for very long, so we shouldn't put the expectation on ourselves that we always need to be completely "into" our sweethearts.

By the way, I noticed at the end of your question you say, "not as desperate to talk to them." I'm not sure if you used the word *desperate* deliberately, but desperation isn't what relationships should be about. Of course we miss our sweeties when we don't see or talk to them, but if we have come to depend on our sweetheart or our relationship to make us feel like a complete person, that's not healthy. Remember, you're two individual people in a relationship, not a relationship of two combined people.

Q: I think I may be in love with two people. Is that possible or just my brain tricking me?

A: First let's talk about the difference between attraction, infatuation, lust, and love.

Attraction is that initial spark that draws us to someone. It's the thing that makes us take a second look. When we are attracted to someone we want to look at them and be around them. Attraction doesn't really depend on knowing them or even talking to them. It's something in us that gets triggered.

Infatuation is having a strong interest in someone. It's thinking about that person a lot (both in sexual and nonsexual ways). It's getting to know a lot about them, either directly or from friends, social media, or whatever. Infatuation often feels like love, but it's almost always one-sided. We are infatuated with someone but, sadly, they're rarely infatuated with us.

Lust is just a physical and sexual attraction. We lust for people whom we want to be with sexually. We don't often think about them as whole people—that can even ruin the lust.

Dr. Ken George, who was one of my graduate school teachers, created one of the best definitions of love I know. He defines love as "best friend + sexual desire."

Given that definition of love, I'd say it's pretty hard to be truly in love with more than one person at a time. We can certainly be attracted to, infatuated with, and even lust for many people at the same time. We can have connections that are intimate and passionate with different people to different degrees, but I think love is pretty special and doesn't usually happen for more than one person at a time.

Now, I do believe people your age can be in love. I don't think it's exactly the same kind of love that you'll be in when you're in your twenties or thirties, but I do believe love between young people is real and powerful. If you are in love with someone, you want to commit fully to that person. Being in love with two people means being fully committed to two people, which seems like a contradiction to me. I'd suggest looking at your feelings again and seeing if you can't figure out what else might be going on here.

Q: Is it possible to be in love with someone and yet have no sexual attraction to them whatsoever? There is someone I think I am in love with. I think about them every second of every day, I live for the time I spend with them, and I would give absolutely anything for them to be happy. Despite such strong feelings, I have no sexual attraction to this person whatsoever. I just don't understand my feelings and am incredibly frustrated!

A: I can understand how frustrating this must feel. I'm glad you asked this question.

There are many different kinds of love—not all of them are sexual. Perhaps what you feel is a deep sense of caring for this person. Is this person destined to be your best friend rather than your sweetheart?

Here's another idea. Perhaps you admire this person so much that you find yourself obsessively thinking about them, but it's more that you want to be *like* them rather than be *with* them.

Another possibility is that you think so highly of this person that you can't imagine them being sexual with anybody. Sometimes we put people on such a high pedestal that we can't imagine them doing something as potentially messy as sex—or we can't imagine that they could possibly want to have sex with us, so we bury any sexual attraction we may feel for them.

Sexual attraction isn't something we can make happen. It's not as if you can make yourself feel something for someone else if you try hard enough. It sounds as though you think you *should* feel sexual attraction for this person. Maybe all that pressure is blocking it from happening.

You may also be someone who's asexual. Asexual people can have deep intimacy and connection with people, but it's not sexual. Asexual people have relationships and sweethearts. Some involve physical interactions like cuddling or touching, or even making out, but not genital sexual activity. Other asexual relationships are strictly platonic and have no physical component. Being asexual or aromantic is just another way to be human.

I'm sorry I can't say for certain what's happening, but I hope you'll consider some of the ideas here.

....

CHAPTER 5

Sex and Gender:
Who's Who and What's What?

After the last few stragglers have stumbled into class, I say, "Have I got a story for you this morning!" This is greeted by a chorus of chatter including:

"Oh, I get nervous when you say that, Mr. V."

"Is it sexy?"

"Do we need to take notes on it, or can we just listen?"

"I was *hoping* there'd be a story today!"

"No notes; this is more of a guided meditation," I say. "All you need to do is close your eyes, if you're so inclined, and listen. We'll talk about the story a bit afterward. As I tell the story, try to put yourself in the place of the main character. What would you be thinking and feeling as the story unfolds? OK, here we go."

"You're making your way through a typical day at school, moving from class to class, and anxiously waiting for lunch. As you finally stroll into the cafeteria and saddle up next to your friends at your usual table, you realize that something is amiss. You check, and, to your surprise and amazement, you find that your genitals are missing! Yes, your penis and scrotum or your vulva just aren't there! You know they were there this morning when you got to school. But sometime between first period and lunch, they just fell off somewhere."

At this point the room erupts in laughter and chatter and (mostly) fake screams of horror.

"But," I continue, trying to quiet the din, "you don't panic because you are a smart, sexy, savvy student in the Sexuality and Society class. You know what to do. You eat a quick lunch and then make your way to the school's Office of Lost and Missing Genitals."

More laughter breaks out in the room. Some kids quip about not waiting to have lunch first; others say it depends on what's on the menu. Some look to their friends for reassurance that genitals don't really just fall off, and if the school actually has an Office for Lost and Missing Genitals.

"You arrive at the office and are greeted by the nice lady sitting behind her desk knitting. You mumble that you've lost something and ask if any genitals have been turned in today.

"She smiles and chuckles a bit. 'Oh my, yes,' she says. 'It's been a big day for lost genitals! Just go in the back, dear, and see if yours is there.' "

"You wander into the back room and are greeted by walls lined with steel-gray shelving. Filling the shelves are all manner of genitals that people have lost. All you have to do is pick up your own, and you're good to go."

I pause a little, let the scenario sink in a bit, and then continue. "So, here's the important question: how likely are you to be able to pick out your own genitals?"

Where you might expect more noise in the class, there's usually just a bit of stunned silence. It's typical that a boy breaks it.

"Duh!" says a tall boy who is filled with self-confidence. "That's easy. I'd just call its name and it would leap into my waiting arms." Yes, lots of teenage (and adult) men name their penises. A few other boys join in and agree that they're 100 percent certain they could find their penis on the shelf. Some other boys are more quiet, which is OK and actually instructive to the boys who are laughing.

I then turn my attention to the rest of the class. "What about you all?"

Often when the young women speak, there is little to no laughter. Most confess that they wouldn't have any idea which vulva is theirs. Many say that they've never seen their own vulva. A few think they can pick out their vulva and seem proud of that. I point out how much the energy level in the room has shifted. The boys stare. Most can't imagine not knowing what their genitals look like.

"For people who are sexually active with a sweetheart," I say, "how would you do picking out their genitals from the shelf?" The tables turn a bit as some of the heterosexual girls say they could pretty confidently pick out their boyfriend's penis, however, few of the heterosexual boys think they would know their sweetheart's vulva. Only a few times have kids who are gay and lesbian spoken up, but they tend to feel more confident about being able to pick out their own or their sweetheart's genitals.

In processing this activity with the students, they make a lot of important points: Penises are more public; men look at and touch them when they urinate and masturbate. Society is pretty quiet about vulvas. It isn't a universal experience for women to be taught to know their vulvas or be proud of them. Many women get negative messages about their vulvas, that they're dirty or smelly. Rather than appreciate the unique beauty and variety of vulvas, some women undergo plastic surgery on their labia to make them "look right." And so our unit on sex and gender begins.

Sex: Who We Are, Not What We Do

Many sexuality education classes, including mine, have lessons on reproductive anatomy and physiology. When done poorly, these lessons amount to little more than labeling diagrams of binary male and female reproductive systems. Even the language, "reproductive systems" or "reproductive anatomy," is troubling to me. Of course those organs and systems are used for reproduction, but that's not what most people use them for most of the time. I always call them the "sexual and reproductive systems," and discuss not only their reproductive capabilities but also their capacities for pleasure, intimate connection, and self-discovery.

It's essential to make the distinction between sex and gender here. When we're talking about biology, we're talking about sex, not sex as a thing people do (a verb), but sex as who people are (a noun). Without a clear understanding of the difference between sex and gender, my students will be ill equipped to have the kind of conversations I want to have in class. So, let's first talk about sex, and then we can talk about gender and the interplay between the two.

Human sexual reproduction, the process of creating a new biological organism, requires a sperm cell and an egg cell. Egg cells carry an X chromosome (usually just one, but on occasion more than one). Sperm cells can carry either an X chromosome or a Y chromosome (usually just one, but on occasion more than one). As soon as sperm meets egg, the combination of chromosomes creates a biological blueprint for our sex (but not our gender). As humans develop there are three paths a body can take: male, female, and intersex. Notice the language here. *Male* and *female* are biological terms. *Man/boy* and *woman/girl* are gender terms. *Intersex* is a word that describes a human being whose biology (whether chromosomally, hormonally, or anatomically) is different from what we think of as a typical male or female body. Intersex people aren't mistakes or aberrations; they're naturally occurring human variations, and there are a lot of them! It's estimated that one in every two thousand births is an intersex person. For context, that's about the same number of people who are redheads. A minority to be sure, but a sizable one. In the past, the word used to describe an intersex person was *hermaphrodite*. We don't use this term now because it's both offensive and inaccurate. Hermaphrodite suggests a mixing of typically male and female characteristics, but that reinforces the false idea that humans *should* be only male or female. This binary thinking, like all binary thinking, is problematic. As we'll see, biologically, male and female are not completely separate entities but more like two points on a vast continuum.

Intersex people can have genetic codes that are different from the XX and XY we're familiar with. They may be XXX, XYY, XXY, XXXY, XO, or even have some cells that are XX and others that are XY in the same body. Their bodies produce estrogen and testosterone to varying levels, and those hormones shape the body's anatomy. Intersex people may develop testes, ovaries, neither of these, or a combined organ called an ovotestis, and in very rare occurrences they can have one fully formed ovary and one fully formed testis. Intersex genitals may look typically male, typically female, like some combination of the two, or unlike any genitals we're familiar with. Some intersex people can reproduce and some can't. When intersex babies are born, parents often face enormous pressure to "correct" their baby's genitals to make them look more like a typical penis and scrotum or vulva, even if the intersex genitals function perfectly well. Others argue that intersex children should be allowed to grow up without any unnecessary surgical intervention until they can decide on their own whether they want to alter their bodies in any way. It's the insistence on seeing sex as a binary, exclusively male or female, that leads to this pressure to make infants' bodies conform to what we think of as more typical. If we could come to appreciate the full range of possibilities of biological sex, we would be more welcoming of intersex babies and adults, and not feel so bound to the artificial binary that our society so rigidly enforces.

As you can see, there are many components that make up our biological sex. It's an interplay among our chromosomes, the way our body makes and uses hormones, our internal and external anatomy, and even the way our brains are constructed. When we're born, we are *assigned* a sex. Usually this assignment is made by taking a cursory look at our genitals. If what's there looks like a penis, we hear "It's a boy!" (more precisely, it should be "It's a male!"). If what's there looks like a vulva, we hear "It's a girl!"

(which really should be "It's a female!"). If what's there doesn't look like either a penis or a vulva, or looks like a combination of both, well, we're still not very good at knowing what to say. (I'd suggest, "It's a beautiful baby!")

We were likely raised with the notion of sex as binary and that male and female bodies are very different. It's often suggested that males can't truly understand the workings of the female body and vice versa. This is ridiculous when you think that most people are heterosexual and good sex depends on our understanding, appreciating, and celebrating each other's bodies. Our binary thinking often paints our sexual and reproductive parts as opposites, and popular magazines are filled with articles with detailed instructions to teach men the intricacies of clitoral stimulation and women the best technique for stimulating a penis. The truth is, though, when it comes to our genitals, we just aren't that different. This is a lesson that always blows my students' minds and their parents' minds when they go home and repeat it around the dinner table.

There's no doubt that male, female, and intersex genitals (the word *genitals* refers to our external sexual organs) look different. But that appearance masks an important biological reality. Human embryos growing in the womb have different genetic makeup, but no matter what their genetic code is, at six weeks of development they all have the same ambiguous blob of tissue between their legs that will become their genitals. Then, according to the blueprint coded in the DNA, the hormones the body develops, and the way that body responds to those hormones, that little blob will shape into a penis and scrotum, a vulva, or something else.

In other words, our genital anatomy, no matter what it looks like, is really the same tissue, just shaped differently. The head of a penis and the clitoris are formed from the same tissue and both provide a focus of sexual pleasure, but since they look different, we often assume that they're alien to each other. The scrotum (the sac that holds the testes) and the labia majora (the outer lips of the vulva) are, again, the same tissue in different form. And the skin of the shaft of the penis and the labia minora, or inner lips, of the vulva are the same tissue, again just shaped differently. Interestingly, ovaries and testes, although internal organs, work like this as well. There's a second blob of embryonic tissue that will become an ovary, a testis, or an ovotestis.

The rest of our internal sexual and reproductive structures do have their own unique origins. There are different embryonic "kits," one programmed to develop into internal female structures (fallopian tubes, a uterus, a vagina) and one programmed to develop into internal male structures (a prostate, vas deferens, Cowper's glands, etc.), but every human embryo, no matter what their genetic code, is equipped with both "kits"! Which kit gets used is determined, again, by our genetic blueprint and hormones. The unused kit just degenerates.

There's a fun way to illustrate how similar genitals are anatomically. It's one of the lessons my kids always remember from the Sexuality and Society class. One day when they come into class I give each of them a can of Play-Doh. After covering a few very important ground rules: no throwing Play-Doh, no eating Play-Doh, and no sticking Play-Doh into each other's hair or clothes, I invite them to mold their Play-Doh into a set of genitals (male, female, or intersex—their choice). This is an invitation, not a requirement;

kids are always allowed to "pass" on any in-class activity that violates their values, although very few kids have ever chosen not to participate over the years. In fact, they giggle and cheer and raise all kinds of ruckus when they set to their task. That noise is important; it allows them to burn off nervous energy.

To some readers this may seem totally off base, but it's actually an important tactile lesson—I'm giving the students permission to touch things that look like genitals for an educational purpose, which makes all of us more comfortable. When they've completed their sculpture, I'll ask them to consider how to turn it into another kind of genital by just reshaping what they've done. They can't crumble everything back into a blob and start over. They'll study it carefully and then reshape the Play-Doh with their hands. It shows them that you really can reshape a scrotum into labia, just by spreading the clay up and outward. When you push the head of the penis back to make it a clitoris, the shaft of the penis opens up to create the inner labia. It's fun to watch their faces, as they discover how cool our bodies are. I'm all about desensitizing and demystifying body parts to help kids understand how their bodies work. One way to do this is to give them numerous ways to explore them safely. Although I do this activity with twelfth-graders, it can be done with any age. It's a nonthreatening way to introduce the genitals.

Given all this information about how our bodies develop, I encourage my students to stop referring to males and females as opposites. How can we be opposite if our bodies are made up of fundamentally the same tissue? In my class we say "other" sex instead of "opposite" sex. This is also important because *opposite* implies two while *other* does not. And we know that humans can be more than just male and female. It's disrespectful and imprecise to use such limited language to explore such a diverse reality.

Lest you think I spend all my time trying to point out how similar males and females are, I do acknowledge and spend time talking about our differences. The next few paragraphs will seem like I'm reverting to the binary. The problem is the glaring lack of widely available studies on intersex bodies. There has been a lot of comparison of male and female bodies, but not enough comparing of those bodies to their intersex counterparts.

I often joke that, biologically speaking, males are built for short, nasty lives, while females are built for long, enduring ones. Put a male and a female next to each other, and it's clear they're physically different. Males tend to be bigger. They have larger upper bodies, giving them lots of upper-body strength, and they tend to be square shaped. Females are curvier. They tend to be shorter. They tend to have stronger lower bodies.

Our constitutions are also very different. We know that, on average, females live longer than males. We know that male babies die more frequently than female babies do. Males are better at using their energy in quick bursts. Females are better at using their energy at a slower pace. They carry and bear children, which requires an incredible amount of physical endurance to be sustained over an extended period of time. Males may be faster runners, but I'd bet on a female's endurance to beat out the male's any day.

Our reproductive strategies are different in fascinating ways. On a strictly biological level, reproduction is a way to ensure that one's genetic material is passed on to the next generation. If you're a female, getting pregnant and giving birth are proof that your genes have made it to the next generation. But if you're a male, what's the guarantee—strictly biologically speaking—that your genes have successfully been passed on? There actually isn't one. So, males produce trillions of sperm cells during their lives and send them out into the world. The more you send out, the more likely it is that one of them will fertilize an egg. Females only use a few hundred egg cells during their fertile lives and tend to release only one egg cell during each menstrual cycle. Since pregnancy and birth are so taxing on the body, you don't want to have too many egg cells available. Males are fertile from puberty until death, giving abundant chances to get sperm into the world. Females have a limited fertility period since pregnancy at too young or too old an age could be threatening to the mother's and child's lives. It's important to remember that we're talking strictly about biology here. This does not mean that males are naturally hornier or more likely to be unfaithful, or that females are more naturally prudish or nurturing. We are more than our biology, and our society likely has much more to do with how we respond (or don't respond) to our reproductive capabilities.

Male and female brains are wired differently. Female brains are much better at memory tasks, while males excel at visual spatial tasks. Females are better at reading and understanding emotions and emotional cues, a particularly helpful skill when caring for a newborn, nonverbal infant. And while females have several areas of the brain that can process language, males have one main area in the brain for that task. This may be one reason why females are more likely to recover language after a stroke than males are.

We need to be careful not to treat biology as destiny here. This is equally important in the classroom and around the dinner table. Yes, generally females are more verbal than males but not always. Male brains may be better attuned to master subjects like geometry, but plenty of them still struggle with it. There's a balance needed between attributing every word and action to biology and ignoring any impact of it. Yes, male, female, and intersex brains think differently, but we can't make those differences restrict what we expect of one another.

We know that these differences are true—research has consistently shown them. But what we don't know, and what we can't know, is how much of this is nature and how much of this is nurture. Humans are and have always been social animals. Those societies we create have a profound impact on our biology, even changing it over time. Take the earliest human communities. The accepted understanding is that labor was divided by hunters and gatherers. Were males hunters because they had better upper-body strength, were more aggressive and better at manipulating objects in space, which made them better able to throw a spear and hit a tiger? Or did males just take on these hunting jobs, and male bodies evolved to make them better hunters? Similarly with females, it made sense that they didn't go out on the hunt if they were pregnant or caring for young children. Were they gatherers because they had such good lower-body strength needed for squatting and picking, and memories that could identify which berry bushes were delicious and which were poisonous—or did a female's memory and lower body sharpen and strengthen because she was expected to know where the best berry bushes were? The point isn't to answer these questions, but to consider how biology and society are so intertwined in making us who we are.

Our focus in this unit is on knowing how our bodies function and feel so that we can be more confident and comfortable with them, and so that we can be more confident and comfortable romantic and sexual partners. My bottom-line message in this unit is always, "You have to be the expert on your own body, you have to know what 'normal' is for your body, and you have to know how your body feels and functions so you can explain it to a partner and they can appreciate its magnificence as much as you do."

But Children Shouldn't Say That, Should They?

Perhaps the thought of using this terminology with your kids might make you uncomfortable. Don't let it. They're just words. Many parents build up a lot of anxiety at the thought of a young child using words like penis, vulva, or intersex. Quick sidenote here, "vulva" is the correct term for a female's external genitals. A vagina is an internal organ. You can't see a vagina when you look at a naked female body; it's inside. The parts you can see are collectively called the vulva.

Too many of my twelfth-graders don't know that, and I've met many adults who don't know it either. How can we be experts on our own bodies if we don't know what our parts are actually called? That brings up a question many parents ask me: "When is it OK to teach a child words like penis and vulva? Isn't it better to give them alternative words for their genitals when they're young?" You'll notice how this question is leading: it contains the answer many parents want me to give them. My answer is always that children should know the correct anatomical names for their genitals from the start. Providing an alternate name for genitals, especially diminutive ones like *pee-pee* or *coochie*, sends messages that children may misinterpret. Kids are smart enough to know that what isn't named—what is coded—is taboo or shameful.

Modesty about one's genitals is always appropriate. Shame about one's genitals is never appropriate. Modesty means one doesn't yell "penis" in a crowded room, but that knowing the word *penis* is not immodest.

Now that we have a better handle on understanding biological sex, we can turn to exploring gender—and that's much more complex than biology!

Exploring Gender from Within and from Without

While sex is strictly biological, gender isn't. I'm not saying there's no connection between sex and gender, but that connection is heavily influenced, and I'd say much more influenced, by culture and sociological forces than by biology. I define gender as "a set of constructed rules or norms that a society assigns to a person based on their assigned sex at birth." So, although there's no strict biological basis for it, our society assumes (and I'm generalizing here) that males are naturally stoic and tough while females are naturally emotional and delicate (and notice the corresponding lack of any generalities about intersex people). Gender is constructed by a society; that's why there are different rules for what's acceptable for people of different sexes in different societies. If gender were strictly biologically based, we wouldn't expect to see such variation in gender expectations around the globe.

Although gender is essentially invented, that doesn't mean it's not important. Gender is one of the most significant lenses we use to examine and make sense of the world. Gender gets *assumed* as soon as birth sex is assigned. Blue and pink receiving blankets often swaddle babies because we assume that male children are boys and female children are girls. Notice the language shift here. When we're talking about gender we should use terms like *man/boy, woman/girl, nonbinary/child*. We're talking about an aspect of identity that is less about the parts a person has and more about the assumptions our society makes about what someone with those parts should do.

Gender is one of the single biggest identity markers in a person's life and understanding our gender identity ultimately changes the way we interact with our bodies and the larger world. *Gender identity* refers to one's internal, personal sense of their own gender. This is something that develops in young children and seems to become pretty solid by age three or four. We don't understand the exact process by which gender identity forms, but it's not strictly biological. It's an interplay between our bodies, our interactions with the world, and some esoteric creation of self that's beyond both of those. I'm not trying to be mysterious here, it's just a process that is not fully understood.

Here's what we can say. Some people, probably the majority of people in today's world, have a gender identity that aligns with their biology, their assigned sex at birth, and with the societal assumptions made about individuals with that biology. This is called being *cisgender*. So, as a cisgender man, I have a male body, was assigned a boy at birth, have always identified and seen myself as a boy/man, and (generally) adhere to the societal expectations assigned to men. Someone whose gender identity does not align with their sex assigned at birth is *transgender*. This is a term that's becoming more normalized but also quite loaded in our society today, but that's because a lot of false assumptions get piled onto that word. At the core, a transgender person's gender identity (their internal, personal sense of self) does not align with the sex they were assigned at birth. It may, but doesn't have to, include a feeling of disconnect with some or all of one's body. It may, but does not have to, include a desire to change one's biological or social appearance so that they will be perceived by the world more as the gender they know themselves to be. We'll get into this more later, but for now it's important to break what seems like the unbreakable link between sex and gender. They're not the same, and we cause harm to people (and maybe to ourselves) when we assume they are.

One more term that's important to understand is *gender expression*. At its most basic, this is how we show the world what gender we are, which can be different from what gender the world assumes we are. Gender is expressed in a huge variety of ways: our clothing, our hairstyle, our body adornment, our hobbies, our professions, our social behaviors, our language choices, our pronouns, and so much more. We put ourselves into the world in deliberate ways so that the world sees us and understands us as we see and understand ourselves. That is, unless we fear the world will not accept us or harm us because of how we see and understand ourselves. Then we might feel like we have to hide ourselves or put ourselves into the world in ways that feel inauthentic, unnatural, or just plain wrong. People don't do this because they want to; they do it to survive, and it's a gross injustice.

Kids (and adults) are constantly being taught powerful lessons about gender expectations through toys, books, clothing, TV, movies, video games, social media, and everything that surrounds them, and many of these messages are OK. I don't want anyone to think I'm arguing that there's something wrong with strongly identifying as a boy or a girl. There's nothing wrong with being a boy who likes sports or a girl who likes dresses—as long as that feels authentic to them.

As we transition from talking about gender as a biological quality to a sociological construct, I use a lesson that the kids love to hate. As they pile into class, I've written seven names on the board. This sparks one of their favorite questions.

"Are we doing an activity today?"

"You bet," I say, and they erupt into cheers and chatter. Once they've settled I give them the instructions. "I'm going to read you a story. The first time I read it I just want you to listen to it. The second time I read it I'll give you specific instructions for what to do with it." Then I read the story just as it's printed below. I point to the character names on the board as they appear in the story. Go ahead, give it a read yourself.

A Day at the Beach

....

Terry's parents were going out of town for the weekend and Terry thought that would provide a great opportunity to have a little party for a few friends. Terry called Chris, Lee, and Sam and invited them to the party. Chris asked if there would be booze at the party. Terry's parents did not drink and had no liquor in the house, but Terry said there would definitely be booze at the party. Terry went to the liquor store, but being underage and having no ID, Terry could not buy the booze. A stranger, Pat, agreed to buy the booze for Terry and charged a $20.00 *"service fee." Terry gladly paid the money and Pat provided the booze. Coach Martin was passing by the liquor store at the time and saw the entire transaction between Terry and Pat. It being summer, the coach ignored the whole situation.*

Later that night, Terry, Lee, Chris, and Sam were at the beach house having a good time. Chris had always thought Lee was hot and decided tonight would be a perfect opportunity to make a move. Chris never let Lee's cup go empty. After an hour or so of drinking, Chris suggested they go upstairs. Sam noticed that Lee looked awfully drunk and that Chris was paying a lot of attention to Lee. Sam followed the pair upstairs and found Lee passed out on the bed. Chris seemed scared and didn't know what to do. Sam told Terry, who made a call to Dr. Green to ask for advice. Dr. Green called 911 and Terry's parents. Lee was taken to the hospital and was released a few hours later perfectly fine. Terry's parents decided on a week's grounding as a punishment for Terry, for having the party and buying booze.

The second time I read the story, I ask the students to assign gender to all the characters.

"Can we use the whole spectrum of gender identity or are we assuming a gender binary?" asks a young woman who's always thinking a bit deeper than the rest of the class.

"Spectrum of what?" ask several other kids.

"You know," the young woman continues. "Could some of the people in the story be transgender, or genderqueer, or things like that."

"She's making things complicated again, Mr. V," several students whine.

"Well, life is complicated," I say. "And we know that people can identify their gender in all kinds of ways. We have members of our community who identify as nonbinary, transgender, or gender diverse. But for this activity let's assume it takes place in a backward universe where a strict gender binary is in place. Your only options for this activity are man/boy and woman/girl."

The kids get to work. The noise level in the room waxes and wanes as they discuss and debate their choices. After about five minutes we start discussing the results. I go through each character and by simple show of hands ask students whether they thought that character was a boy or a girl. After we finish, the students only want to know one thing.

"Did we get it right?"

If I tell them now that there are no right or wrong answers and the activity only reveals their assumptions about gender, they'll lose interest, so I string them along in that tried-and-true teacher fashion.

"Before I tell you that, I want to hear some rationale for your choices. I want to make sure you really knew the right answers and didn't just guess."

Challenge accepted. They have a million different reasons why they labeled a character as a boy or a girl. They talk about which characters were hard to figure out and which were easy. Coach Martin almost always gets labeled as a guy. Chris and Lee are usually assigned as a heterosexual couple: Chris boy and Lee girl. Sam is a toss-up, depending on the motivation for following Chris and Lee upstairs—a boy might do it to cheer on his "bro"; a girl might do it to check up on her girlfriend. Terry's gender generates the most discussion. Some think she's a girl, because she asks someone to get the booze for her and because of what the students see as a lenient punishment given by her parents. Others argue that Terry must be a boy, sometimes for the very same reasons. Dr. Green is always a hard character to decide because they do what any doctor should do no matter their gender. As we near the end of the class, the students return insistently to their earlier question—"Did we get it right??" they beg.

They, of course, cry foul when I tell them there are no right or wrong answers. I point out how there are no biological gender markers for any character in the story. The only things the students had to use in assigning gender were the characters' personality traits, attitudes, and actions, and, in truth, the students were really relying on *their own* gender identity and assumptions about the characters' behavior. It's an activity that is much more about them than about the fictional characters in the story.

"You got us again, Mr. V," says a boy who high-fives me as he walks out of class.

Gender Scripts: Roles, Rules, and (Often Stifling) Expectations

Gender roles, or *gender scripts*, are culturally constructed codes of behavior for how a person is supposed to behave in a society given their gender. They're not about individuality and uniqueness; they're about pinning things down, delineating one gender from another, and keeping people in line. They're about maintaining privilege and power. That's not to say they're always problematic. There's a lot of benefit a society gains from having clear expectations for behavior. It certainly makes it easier to navigate day-to-day life. The problems with gender scripts come when we forget they are societal constructions and start to believe they are somehow immutable, and when they become so rigid that they stifle individuality and authenticity. How a society creates and reinforces its gender roles has a lot to do with the overall sexual health of the society. Societies with the strictest gender scripts have more sexual assault, more child sexual abuse, more violence against women, and more homophobia and transphobia.

Gender scripts influence what we wear and how we talk and interact with other people, and when someone does something that violates our ideas about gender, which I call a *gender violation* or *gender foul*, it can make many people uncomfortable. Gender scripts care more about outward appearance than internal consistency. If an individual doesn't want to conform to a society's gender scripts it's often assumed there's a problem with them, not with the scripts. They have to get in line. If we assume that gender expression is a binary continuum with the most macho man at one end and the girliest of girls on the other, how far into the middle can you go before it's considered a gender violation? Can a boy read *Cosmo* and retain his manhood? If a girl puts pressure on her boyfriend to have sex, is she still a girl? What if she openly burps and farts? When is crying acceptable for a man? When is it a foul? What are the accepted gender scripts for someone who doesn't subscribe to binary gender? What's expected of nonbinary or gender-diverse people?

What's acceptable on the gender front is determined not only by the macro society in which we live, but also by our micro communities: where we go to school, our ethnic heritage, and the group of people we're with. For example, what's allowable for a guy at dinner with his sweetheart may be different from what his teammates let slide on the soccer team. A frequent discussion in my class is who has more leeway in terms of gender expression: boys, girls, or nonbinary people? Girls readily admit that they can wear much more masculine clothing and participate in traditionally boy activities (e.g., chess team, science clubs, math team) without losing their girlness. Heterosexual boys will tell me that they live by stricter gender scripts than heterosexual girls or gay boys do, especially because they're beyond terrified of being perceived as gay. For boys, certain colors are off-limits when it comes to clothing. Some cars are too feminine to drive, some drinks or foods too "girly" to consume. Nonbinary students often face a world who wants to push them into a box they're intentionally trying to avoid. Because so many gender scripts are based on the binary, people often don't know how to react when someone steps outside of it.

The popularity of bromance movies has helped stage what physical interactions are OK for two boys in terms of relating to each other emotionally, and which are not. Boys can joke about a relationship between two boys being sexual, but only when there's a very clear understanding that it's not. Two heterosexual boys are allowed to hug, as long as they pound each other on the back. They're allowed to do complicated, touchy handshakes as long as they finish it off with a chest bump. They're allowed to be sexual with each other as long as they keep their socks on. (I don't understand that one either, but it's apparently a rule.) Boys share a lot of intimacy, but it's rare for them to talk about their emotions directly. Often they're drunk or in crisis when those topics emerge.

Girls are often portrayed as freer with their emotions—can you imagine a breakup scene in a movie where the girl *didn't* cry or get angry? They snuggle in the same bed during sleepover parties, and they often hug or tell each other how important they are to one another. They don't obviously cross gender lines until they do something extreme like shave their head. That might be a societal assumption, but my students tell me that's not necessarily true. Gender foul is called on girls frequently. It just happens to be more about violating the girl code of being a "good girl" or "nice girl" or "pretty girl." Since being perceived as sexually promiscuous is often seen as a gender foul for girls, they cry foul if a girl dates her good friend's ex-boyfriend. If a girl cheats on her boyfriend or even goes too far "too soon" with her current guy, she'll be deemed a slut.

My gender-diverse and nonbinary students sometimes tell stories of complete invisibility—people refuse to see or acknowledge them. People ignore their names and pronouns and try to force them into a box that makes it "easier" for society. On the other hand, sometimes they tell stories of great freedom. Once they step outside of the gender binary, they are able to construct a self that truly fits who they are on the inside. It takes enormous strength of will to stand outside of the box, especially as an adolescent.

Their strength is having an important impact on our society. My students today are so much more comfortable with transgender, nonbinary, and gender-diverse folks than they were fifteen years ago. They are more willing to question the rigid, often suffocating roles society insists on for gender conformity. They are more able to understand that gender fouls are often a case of sexism and heterosexism. They're power plays designed to keep men, and more specifically straight men, in charge.

I encourage students to think about who really benefits from policing gender. As I said earlier, a general sense of boundaries can benefit all of us, but the rigid enforcement that limits gender roles for men and women and ignores others outside of the gender binary squashes individuality and can inhibit the expression of our authentic selves. I'm sure we've all experienced a time when we checked our own behaviors or reactions because they didn't seem correct for our gender. There are other times when we've blown past any delineated lines. Even when acknowledging this, it can be scary for kids to question any of the assumptions society makes about gender.

When a coach calls the boys on his team "ladies" as a way to make them work harder, it takes a lot of courage to call him on it. When a girl is called a "whore" because she's sexually active in ways that go against what's seen as appropriate for her gender, who sticks up for her? It's vitally important that my students understand that they, and only they, are the arbiters of what their gender means to them. They are the ones who can decide how much to conform to the gender scripts that are handed to them at every turn—and those decisions are best when they honor their authentic selves. As I said before, there's nothing wrong with a guy liking sports or a girl liking fashion as long as it's because that's who they really are and not because that's who they think they're supposed to be.

So, it's OK that we've created rules and roles about how we behave gender-wise. It would be pretty confusing without them. It's only bad if those roles and rules get so rigid that we have to stop being our authentic self to fit into a prescribed notion of what our gender looks like. When kids are given the tools to under-stand the way that gender assumptions play into their decisions, they may begin to follow their own inner compass, instead of doing what they think they should do.

Pronouns and Labels—Why All the Fuss?

I've always been an English teacher as well as a sexuality educator, which means I care about language and have great respect for proper grammar and usage. When people hear that, they can assume I'm bothered by the use of *they* and *them* as singular pronouns. I'm not. First of all, the singular *they* has been part of the English language for a long time. The *Oxford English Dictionary* traces its first use back to 1375 in the medieval romance *William and the Werewolf*. We may not realize it, but we're already totally comfortable using the singular *they* in English when we don't know the gender or sex of the person we're talking about. For example, think about how natural this sentence sounds: "Someone left their umbrella in the classroom. I hope they come and get it before the thunderstorms start." So, let's stop arguing grammar and get to the real heart of the matter.

One of the biggest changes I've seen in young people from when I started teaching is their comfort with the fluidity of identity and the labels they use to describe their genders. Back in the "old days," identity was something assumed by most to be fixed. You were born into a body, which assumed your gender, which conformed to the rules set forth by your society. End of story. But as we've come to be more understanding of the differences between sex, gender, and sexual orientation—and as our society has gotten more comfortable with moving beyond all kinds of binaries—young people's understanding of identity development has shifted.

Young people know they are living in a world with a huge

variety of options for how to describe themselves. They are not limited to a few rigid labels. When it comes to gender identity, kids may identify as: boy, girl, nonbinary, demiboy, demigirl, agender, gender fluid, genderqueer, gender nonconforming, AFAB (assigned female at birth), AMAB (assigned male at birth), pangender, neutrois, two-spirit, and many others. It's not important for you to know every possible gender identity label your kid may present to you—that's an impossible task as new labels come to light all the time. It is essential to know that it's absolutely normal for lots of young people to feel very comfortable trying on different labels at different times in their development. This is a good thing! They have options and there's nothing wrong with exploring them to find which speaks truth to them. Remember, the goal is to determine who they are most authentically. That's a big and important task, and it is aided by the variety of language that's developed to denote differences in gender beyond the binary.

When a young person tells you how they're identifying I suggest, first, to thank them for letting you know. If you haven't heard the term they're using, ask them to explain or define it for you. This isn't a time for interrogation ("Are you sure?") or accusation ("Did that wacky teacher tell you to use that label?"). Your kid is giving you information—that's all. Information is good. I always say to kids, "I'm glad you've found a label that fits. I want you to know that you don't have to make any final declarations today. If this label continues to fit and becomes more true for you, great. If it changes, that's fine too. You're in charge of your identity. I just want to make sure you're being true to yourself."

This past year in our lower school we had a small group of kids who began to use "they/them" pronouns rather than the traditional "he/she" pronouns they had been using. Parents wondered what this meant and if it should be a cause for concern. I didn't think it was and suggested we simply pause, breathe, and see where it went. The teachers and parents were terrific at working to honor the kids' pronouns. They weren't perfect, but perfection isn't the goal. In a couple of weeks something interesting happened. Many of the kids who had been trying out the "they/them" pronouns decided that wasn't actually for them and went back to more traditionally gendered pronouns. A few kids found that "they/them" worked for them and kept using them. The result was kids working to discover what felt most right for them. Yes, even lower school kids can do this.

I understand that it may come as a shock when your kid comes home and announces a new gender identity label or a new set of pronouns they want to use. I can only ask you to pause, breathe, and remember the goal—authenticity. As much as we love the kids in our lives, we can't tell them who they most truly are—only they can do that. We can support that process or we can impede it. I urge you to choose support.

Gender and Sexual Activity: Breaking Down Assumptions About Doing It

I had a female student a few years ago who openly admitted she enjoyed sex for its own sake. "The way guys do," she told me. In that one line, she turned a few gender stereotypes on their head. It's assumed that boys like (and want) sexual activity—they don't always need emotional intimacy to enjoy it. It's also assumed that girls require more emotional intimacy with sexual activity. This is true for some people, but not all. It's just another example of rigid gender scripts. Why are girls thought to "lose" something when having sex? Instead of "losing their virginity," couldn't they be gaining sexual pleasure and fulfillment? What do boys lose when they have sex? Nothing but the stigma of being a guy who hasn't "gotten any." I do think it's important for kids to see that sexual activity and relationships are filled with gender expectations that decrease the chance it will be equitable and physically fulfilling for them.

Oral sex is a great example to use when discussing how gender scripts impact sexual activity. Just so we're clear, a generation ago, oral sex was considered more intimate than sexual intercourse, but today, kids often experience it before they even consider having intercourse. And more, according to today's gender scripts for oral sex, girls are expected to give it without much thought of reciprocation of any kind. When I suggest that I find this situation completely inequitable, the boys in my class get mad at me; they accuse me of violating some kind of "bro code." "It's totally fair," the guys will argue. "Girls like doing it and even if they don't, they do get something out of it—status." The girls often have a huge Aha! moment here, and the brave ones will speak up and bust the myth that all girls like doing it or argue that status and physical pleasure are not equivalent—and that "status" isn't always the badge of honor some boys make it seem.

See, the thing about gender scripts is that they can become so insidious that we stop seeing them. Straight girls think it's a very normal part of the teenage years to give a boyfriend a blow job. But they don't expect a straight boy to perform oral sex on them, or expect that they will receive any kind of sexual pleasure back. This is not to say that girls necessarily want boys to perform oral sex on them, and those that would may be embarrassed to ask—again, all because of what gender scripts tell us about what sexual activity *should* be. The important thing to note is that this really *isn't* about sex. It's about power. I tell my students just to picture the position of people's bodies during oral sex, especially the way they have it. Usually the person receiving oral sex is dominant and the person performing it is submissive. Boys get pleasure, girls give pleasure. But isn't one of the purposes of sexual activity shared pleasure? One of my refrains to the class whenever we talk about sexual activity is, "If you're not as concerned about the other person's pleasure as you are about your own, are you really having sex or are you just using the other person as a glorified masturbation tool?"

Gender scripts exert a powerful pull on our ideas about sexual activity and we buy into them unless we can recognize that they are created constructs, not biological destiny. This is one of the most powerful conversations we can have with young people. It's not about encouraging or discouraging sexual activity; it's about encouraging equity and authenticity. It's about taking charge of what kind of person you want to be.

What Students See When They Look at Gender

At the end of the gender unit comes one of the major assignments of the year. It's called simply "The Gender Project." Students choose some aspect of their lives and design a way to study it specifically through the lens of gender. They can look at just about anything. The only restriction is that they are not allowed to examine their own or others' sexual activity. They can work alone or in groups as they design a research question, collect data, analyze it, and prepare a presentation to share their findings with the class.

After spending many weeks talking about gender as both a biological and a sociological construct, they are primed for this task and they jump into it with gusto. Over the years students have created amazingly diverse and interesting projects. Their results show how much gender impacts every aspect of our lives, and how savvy they have become at seeing it. I thought it might be fun to include a "Top 10" list of favorite Gender Projects over the years. Any of these would be great fodder for a conversation with young people about gender, or you might be inspired to create your own gender project with your kids.

1. Disney Movies from *Snow White* to *Aladdin*: Times Change, Gender Roles Don't

2. "Are You Gonna' Eat That?" An Examination of What Different-Gendered People Buy for Lunch in the School Cafeteria

3. An Examination of Cooking Shows Hosted by Male and Female Chefs on the Food Network: What They Cook, What They Wear, and What Kind of Pots, Pans, and Equipment They Use

4. This Is *Really* Scary: Examining the Differences Between How Men and Women Are Killed in Horror Movies

5. Turkey, Football, and Who Does the Dishes: An Examination of Gender Scripts at My Family's Thanksgiving Dinner

6. Examining Voice-Overs in Commercials: What Male Voices vs. Female Voices vs. Androgynous Voices Are Used to Sell

7. "May I Help You? . . . But Maybe Not You": How the Same Male Salesperson Treats Three Young Women Who Are Dressed Very Differently

8. Examining Gender in *Battlestar Galactica*: In the Future, Women Smoke Cigars

9. Superheroes, Costumes and Gender: Sturdy, Sexy, and Just Plain Scandalous!

10. Lost and Found: What Happens When a Young Man vs. a Young Woman Ask for Directions from Strangers

....

Question Box

Q: I'm a girl, and I hate it when people, even girls, say the word *bitch* to each other or to girls. I don't want to sound rude, but I don't think it's right. What to do?

A: Good for you for wanting to stand up for what you believe is right! There are a couple of ways to handle this situation. I think the best would be to say to someone, "I'm really uncomfortable when I hear that word. Could you not use it when I'm around, please?" Notice how that's an "I statement." It's not saying, "*You're* a bad person because you say that word"; it's expressing your desire not to hear it—which is a completely reasonable thing to request. You could also say something less formal like, "Uh, I hate that word. It's so uncool"—or say whatever feels the most natural to you. Just make it an "I statement."

If someone challenges you on this and asks why you don't like the word, you don't have to give an answer to that, but perhaps it's good to think about why you don't like it. Do you think it demeans women (or men)? Do you think it's disrespectful? Do you think it's crude? Whatever your reason, you're welcome to share it when you ask people not to use the word. You don't have to do that, but sometimes it helps people understand where you're coming from. You might even consider going online and doing some research on the origins and use of the word. You might find support for your view that you can share when talking about it with others.

Q: Is it wrong to assume someone is a man or a woman by their physical appearance?

A: Gender is such an important lens through which we view the world that we can hardly help looking at someone and instantly thinking "man" or "woman." There's nothing wrong with that. Where we get into trouble is when we are not willing to go further than our instantaneous assumptions. We know that gender is not just two boxes labeled "man" and "woman" but a continuum that expresses these ends but also a lot more. Are we willing to go beyond or challenge our initial assumptions or judgments? Are we willing to ask if we don't know? (And, by the way, can we ever actually know for sure unless we ask—aren't we just making an assumption that turns out to be right?) Are we open to an answer that might not be the expected? An important part of respecting a person as an individual is letting them define who they are. It's wrong to shove people into rigid boxes just to make ourselves feel more comfortable. It's not the initial assumption that's the problem; it's what we do after making that initial assumption that counts.

Q: What does society say when girls lose their virginity as opposed to boys?

A: The first thing I want to say about this question is beware what "society" says about any issues involving human sexuality. We live in a pretty sexually unhealthy society in this country, and often the messages that are put out are not helpful in the development of healthy sexuality. Be sure to examine all messages with a critical and analytic eye.

Society makes a distinction about how and when a girl loses her virginity. If she does it on her wedding night, or as part of a loving, stable relationship, society might not have anything bad to say about it. But if a girl loses her virginity in a random sexual encounter or not in the context of a relationship, society is, sadly, likely to look down on her. This furthers the sexist myth that there are "good girls" and "bad girls" and that boys should want to date "bad girls" but marry "good girls." Can you see how this puts both women and men in a no-win situation?

Of course when a boy loses his virginity, no matter how it happens (as long as it's with a woman, that is) he's to be congratulated. How can we help develop healthy sexuality in people when boys are told they *should* lose their virginity and girls are told they *shouldn't*?

The decision about when and how to lose one's virginity is a highly personal decision—one that needs to be made based on

what's best for the individual him/her/themself and their own
values, and not what society tell us.

Q: Do cougars play the field or the game?

A: I assume by "cougar" you're referring to an older woman
who seeks out younger men for sexual partners (usually someone
eight or more years younger than they are). Let's stop and think
about this terminology a bit. If a man seeks out younger partners
is he given such a label? What's the assumption being made
about a woman by calling her a "cougar"? Personally, I see a lot
of sexism and disrespect going on here.

In terms of your question, part of the "cougar" stereotype is
that the woman would be the aggressor (the "pitcher" or "player"
in the baseball model). According to the pizza model, though,
these roles don't mean anything. Either partner can be more aggressive or more passive at any time depending on what they are
feeling. Remember, those baseball rules only exist to restrict and
limit our choices. I'd get rid of the whole "cougar" idea if I were
you. It'll lead to a healthier outlook on sexuality.

CHAPTER 6

....

Sexual Orientation:
Attractions and Actions

"OK, gang, we've got a new topic today, so let's start with an activity!"

The cheers go up around the room: "Yay!"

"Thank God," one sleepy young man says. "I'm too tired to learn anything today." Awake enough to realize what he just said, he looks up at me with a sheepish smile. I give him a quick "you-did-not-just-say-that" look and continue.

"This is called a forced-choice activity," I say. "I'll read a statement and give you four possible answers. Each answer will correspond to a different corner of the classroom. You will move to the corner of the classroom that corresponds with the answer you choose. No standing in the middle of two answers; you've got to pick one of them."

"Wait! We have to *get up and move*?" the same sleepy young man groans. He's not the only one. It's early in the day and nothing is more lethargic than a teenager in the morning.

"Yes, you have to get up and move, but once you move to the

corner that corresponds to your answer, you can sit down," I say, trying to make this a little more palatable.

"I may just crawl." The sleepy boy yawns.

"Mr. V," a young woman in a tight ponytail pipes up, "I don't like this idea of being forced to make a choice! What if it's a really hard question or, like, a really personal one?"

"Not to worry," I say. "One of the possible answers will be 'I don't know.' You can go to that corner of the room if you genuinely don't know the answer, if you simply don't want to answer that question, or if you're just too tired to think." I look over at the sleepy boy, who lifts his head up off of his desk and gives me a weak thumbs-up. "The 'I don't know' corner is a safe zone," I continue. "If you go there, no one can ask you why you're there, and you don't have to answer any questions or make any comments. You'll just be an observer.

"OK, here's the question. Sexual orientation is most likely the result of . . ." I point to one corner of the room. "Biological factors beyond one's control." I point to another corner. "Environmental factors in a person's early life." I point to the third corner and say, "A deliberate choice of the individual." I point to the fourth corner. "I don't know." The students sit there and look at me. *Move!* I shout, and they scatter.

"Can I stand in the middle of two choices?" a girl asks me uncertainly.

"No. Pick a corner!" her friend yells. "Geez, weren't you listening?"

After the groups have settled into their respective corners, I invite a few of the students to talk about why they chose the answer they did. There are always plenty of kids who do, especially if it means arguing with their friends, who might be standing in a different corner.

Kids in the biology corner often say they just believe people are born gay . . . and then someone always starts singing Lady Gaga's "Born This Way." Others in the biology corner cite hearing studies of identical twins that suggested if one is gay their twin has a much higher than average rate of being gay as well. Kids in the environmental corner talk about the early impact of parenting and even bring up the possibility of chemicals in the environment that may cause someone to be gay. Kids in the choice corner often cite people who entered into heterosexual relationships early in life and then divorced and chose to go into a same-gender relationship and call themselves gay.

As the students give their wide-ranging answers, what I'm actually listening for is *whom* they're talking about, not the rationale for their choice. Nearly every time I do this activity, the same thing happens.

"Thanks for your responses, gang," I say. "Before we address them further, I'm interested in seeing if any of you noticed a common feature running through all your responses, no matter what corner you stood in?"

I either get a lot of blank stares or a flurry of off-the-cuff ideas that range from the sublime to the ridiculous.

"That we're all right?"

"That we're all wrong?"

"That we're all awesome?"

"That we're all OK with gay people?"

"Ah! Think about that last comment," I say. "The question was about the cause of sexual orientation, but that isn't exactly the question you answered, was it?"

"Sure it was," a young man in a baseball cap says. "We answered what we think makes people gay."

"So sexual orientation equals gay or not?" I ask.

"Doesn't it?" he asks back.

"No. A more accurate definition is 'an enduring sexual and/or romantic attraction to individuals of a particular gender.'"

"Huh?" he asks, clearly lost in the wording.

"It's whom you fall in love with and in most cases whom you want to have sex with."

"Got it!" he says.

"Can I stick with asking you questions for a minute?" I ask. The young man nods. "Do you have a sexual orientation?"

"I'm not gay," he says.

"Right, I know that," I say. "But that's not the question. Do you have a sexual orientation?"

He doesn't answer right away; he's looking a little puzzled. Finally his girlfriend, who is also in the class, chimes in.

"Um . . . hi, you're straight," she says, blowing him a kiss. He blushes a bit and agrees.

"And which of the factors—biological, environmental, or choice—do you think is most responsible for making you straight?" I ask.

"I dunno. I never thought about it," he says. "Is that wrong?"

"No, it's not wrong at all, but it *is* pretty common. The question I asked was about the root cause of sexual orientation. The question you, and many in the class, answered is about the root cause of homosexuality, but that's just one of any number of possible sexual orientations. The answer you choose should be consistent whether we're talking about what makes a person gay, straight, lesbian, bisexual, or any other orientation."

The class is looking at one another in a way that suggests I've just turned their thinking on its head. Another young man, the once sleepy but now pretty alert one, asks, "So what does make straight people straight?"

"Let's find out," I say. "Now we're ready to start the sexual orientation unit."

Understanding Your Child's Sexual Orientation . . . and Maybe Your Own

One of my core values about sexual orientation is that all orientations are equally valid and should be treated the same. I don't see heterosexuality as any more natural, moral, or important than other orientations, although it is more common. People having a different core value about orientation will see things differently, of course.

As an educator, I teach an integrated approach to sexual orientation. That means my classroom and my curriculum are inclusive of all sexual orientations and gender identities. Quick review of terms here: *gender identity* is our internal sense of our own gender. It's who we "feel" we are at our core and how we label our own gender. *Gender expression* is the external manifestation of our gender identity. It's how we express our gender to the world. We do this through our clothing, language, behavior, preferences, etc.

Sexual orientation is different from gender. I can't stress that point firmly enough. Knowing something about someone's gender does not necessarily tell you anything about their sexual orientation. Gender is about who we are. Sexual orientation is about who we are attracted to. Who we are is certainly connected to that, but does not determine it. Here are a few concrete examples:

I identify as a man and my gender expression is masculine. I am sexually and romantically attracted to people who also identify as men and whose gender expression is masculine. The label I use for my sexual orientation is gay.

One of my friends identifies as a woman and has a feminine gender expression. She finds herself sexually and romantically attracted to people whose gender identity and expression are traditionally men *and* those whose gender identity and expression are traditionally women. She identifies herself as bisexual.

A young person I taught a few years ago who is now in college defines his gender identity as queer. He uses masculine pronouns to describe himself. His gender expression is fluid, ranging from strongly masculine to strongly feminine to all points in between (and, no, his pronoun choice doesn't change based upon his gender expression—he always refers to himself with male pronouns). His sexual and romantic attractions span the gender identity and gender expression spectrum, including people who identify as men, women, transgender, queer, and more. He labels his sexual orientation as pansexual, meaning his attractions cannot be categorized by any particular gender identity.

If this seems confusing to you, why not ask your child about it?

Today's younger generation usually has a better handle on all this. They see gender and sexual orientation as more fluid and less restrictive. Besides, they'd love any opportunity to be *your* teacher. So even if you *do* understand all this, why not play dumb and let your child explain it to you anyway? It might be an "in" to other conversations. As with gender, it's not important for you to know every possible sexual orientation label, but it is important for you to be open to the reality that sexual orientation can be described in ways you probably never thought about, and that's OK.

Remember, gender and sexual orientation are not the same thing, and knowing someone's *gender* identity and *gender* expression does not necessarily mean that you know that person's *sexual orientation*. Oftentimes assumptions are made about a person's sexual orientation based on his or her gender identity and expression. But it's unfair and disrespectful to assume, for example, that your son whose gender expression is masculine is attracted to women and therefore heterosexual. And just because your daughter's gender expression is masculine doesn't mean she's a lesbian. There's only one way to be certain about someone's sexual orientation. You have to ask them! You see, sexual orientation is an *internally applied label*. No one can assign a sexual orientation to another person, and the only valid sexual orientation labels are the ones we give ourselves. And that's why it's so important to teach our kids—all of them—about sexual orientation. We can't truly know who they are until they tell us, and *they* can't know it until they have the chance to learn about it and think about it.

One of the ironic shortcomings of some sexuality education classes today is that they are very open to the wide diversity of sexual orientation, but they often don't give enough, if any, attention to heterosexuality. This robs heterosexual kids of the chance to think about their own journeys and experiences with sexual and romantic attractions. It also creates the false idea for heterosexuals that sexual orientation is about "other" people (non-heterosexuals). My students are always intrigued when I present sexual orientation in a way that's inclusive of heterosexuality. It's a typical Aha! moment, when they consider something they've missed before. They see themselves connected to the content we're studying in a whole new way. I recall one heterosexual student remarking, "I never knew I had a sexual orientation! I thought it was only something gay people had!" Of course there are also students who *have* thought about this before and are surprised when their friends see it as a moment of discovery. In both cases, kids are more ready to engage with the topic, which will lead them to better understanding themselves. It's a total win-win.

For your child, discovering his or her sexual orientation may be a lifelong, evolving process, or perhaps it'll be a quick and easy one. It's important that we give young people the space to talk about their own sexual orientation without judgment, and to help them understand that they don't have to fit into any one label, if that's something they are struggling with. We also need to remind them to extend that courtesy to the other kids around them. This can help stem the tide of bullying around gender and sexual orientation that is happening in too many schools today. Kids of every identity and orientation can be harassed because of assumptions and judgments based on an inaccurate or incomplete understanding of sexual orientation. Talking about this is one of the ways we make schools safer for all kids! Remind them that the label we apply to ourselves today may remain true throughout the rest of our lives, or as our understanding of ourselves changes, that label might change as well. While some young people might stick to commonly understood labels like heterosexual (straight), homosexual (gay/lesbian), and bisexual (bi), there are plenty of others, such as pansexual or omnisexual (attracted to all gender identities and expressions), asexual (having little or no natural sexual or romantic attraction to anyone), demisexual (developing sexual or romantic attraction only after establishing a strong emotional connection), queer (not straight but otherwise not defined by the other labels), MSM (man having sex with men but not identifying as gay or bisexual), and WSW (woman having sex with women but not identifying as lesbian or bisexual).

Transgender is often listed as a sexual orientation, but that isn't exactly accurate. Transgender is a label used by people whose sex assignment at birth is different than their understanding of their own gender identity. It doesn't necessarily mean that a person is "trapped in the wrong body." It just means that the initial, cursory look at a person's physical body as an infant and their internal sense of identity don't match in some way. Some transgender people will alter their physical appearance to bring it more in line with their internal sense of self. This may be reflected in anything from clothing and hairstyle choices to chemically altering one's body with hormones to surgically altering one's body. Some transgender people will alter their pronoun usage, choosing one that best reflects their sense of themselves. Some transgender people don't do any of these things.

Finally, an orientation label that some young people are using today is "questioning." This means exactly what it says, that a person is in the process of figuring out her or his orientation.

It doesn't exclude any answer nor does it imply any answer. It's tricky to say what a questioning kid will look like. Some may experiment with sexual and romantic activity with others; and some will refrain from any such activity until they feel surer of their own identity. Just like with any fundamental question about life, some of us ask it loudly and others prefer a quieter approach. The important thing to note is that most of the kids I've known who identify as questioning aren't anxious about that label. It can be a relief because it means they don't have to apply a label right now and they're open to taking their time to see what label emerges.

....

It is not uncommon for my students to talk to me about their sexual orientation, especially if they are feeling confused. A ninth-grade girl in ripped jeans and a rock band T-shirt came into my classroom one day and asked if we could talk.

"I want to figure out if I'm bi or not," she said matter-of-factly.

"Well," I said, "I'm not the one who can tell you that, but I'm happy to talk with you and listen to your thoughts."

She told me she had been in love with a boy and had a somewhat sexual but definitely romantic relationship with him all during eighth grade. The relationship included making out and some touching of each other's genitals (she burst into peals of laughter when I called that petting). They made a mutual decision to break up upon entering high school. Now she was finding herself sexually and romantically attracted to boys but also to some of her female friends. She knew that what she felt for her eighth-grade boyfriend was real, and she felt sure that these new feelings for girls were real too.

"I'm OK with being bi or even lesbian, if that's what I really am," she said. "I just want to be sure before I go telling people that. So, how do I know?"

"Do you think either the label bisexual or lesbian feels like it fits you right now?" I asked.

"Probably bisexual, if anything," she said.

"Is being bisexual an OK thing according to your values?"

"Yeah," she said. "Whatever I am is OK, and I know it'll be OK with my parents and my friends. I've talked to my parents about this, and they suggested I come talk to you. I'm not freaked out or anything, Mr. V. I'm just trying to figure it out."

"I can see you're not freaked out, and I'm really glad you've talked with your parents and they don't seem freaked out. I heard a possible answer to your question in what you just said. You're trying to figure it out. That seems to be the most appropriate way to describe your orientation right now. You're clearly open to whatever answer is going to emerge, but I don't hear a clear answer now. Do you?"

"No," she said. "So what am I? Bi-curious? Confused?"

"I wouldn't say you're confused; you don't sound confused to me. You sound like you're in a process of discovery. When we're in that kind of process, I think the best we can do is stay open to the possibilities and see what truth emerges over time. If you feel you need to give yourself a label, you also have to be OK with the idea that it's a 'for-now' label. It may shift—or it may not. You need more data. How about 'questioning'? Does that fit?"

"No, because for me it's not a wide-open question; it's more of a fine-tuning. What if I said right now I feel bisexual?"

"Great. I think the most important thing is the 'right now.' Whatever answer you give to yourself and others has to acknowledge that all this is a process and you're interested in find-ing out what's right for you."

This young woman was more open and at ease than other kids who have come to see me, but I think she provides a great exam-ple of how understanding one's own sexual orientation is a lot easier when adults are committed to helping young people find the truth about themselves rather than forcing a label on them. Some kids know the truth about themselves right from the start. Others need time and experience to figure it out. Some people change the label that they use to describe their orientation as they go through life. That's not because their orientation has changed; it's because their understanding or awareness of their orientation changed. The process of discovering one's orientation must be open and patient in order to ultimately be successful. The truth will emerge in its own time. So how do we, as adults, help kids facilitate a process like that? There are lots of ways, and they're all pretty simple.

First, check your own assumptions about a child's sexual ori-entation. You may have a preference for your child's orientation. You may have a value system that makes only some orientations acceptable. That's all fine, as long as you also realize that you (or I or the school or the religious organization or the government) are *not* in charge of creating your child's sexual orientation. Orientations aren't created; they're discovered. And holding that in our minds and hearts is the first way we can help young people.

Second, check your language for assumptions about sexual ori-entation. Imagine yourself saying to your young child, "Someday you'll fall in love with a sweetheart, and it'll be wonderful!" Go further and say, "Sweethearts are people who love each other and want to make a family together." Can you get in the habit of asking children (and even adults, for that matter), "Do you have a sweetheart?" versus asking a girl, "Do you have a boyfriend?" or a boy, "Do you have a girlfriend?" When one of my friends was a teenager, his mother asked him, "When you finally bring a date home for me to meet, is it going to be a girl, or a boy, or what?" My friend matter-of-factly said, "A boy." His mom said, "OK," and that was it. No drama, no long discussion—just a simple question with a simple answer. Our use of language is a way to signal respect and acceptance for all orientations, including the one waiting to be discovered in one's own child.

Third, allow your child (and yourself) to see varied examples of sexual orientation in media, literature, and life. This, of course, should be age appropriate. There are a whole host of children's books, adolescents' novels, and television shows these days that include nonheterosexual characters. There are any number of news events, commercials, and magazine articles that reference people with diverse sexual orientations. There are so many important historical figures who were not heterosexual. Don't be afraid to make that known, and make that just one of many pieces of information you share about the historical figure. It's just as disrespectful to isolate people's sexual orientation as the *only* important thing about them as it is to dismiss their sexual orientation as having no value to what makes them who they are.

Coming Out

Coming out is the process of acknowledging to oneself and then to others one's sexual orientation. Because I teach an integrated approach to this topic, I think coming out as a heterosexual is just as worthy of attention as any other coming-out experience. Not only do I think it is valuable in itself for heterosexuals to consider their own coming out, but I believe it helps them better understand the coming-out experiences of those who aren't heterosexual. I also believe that straight parents who have a child coming out as something other than heterosexual will be better prepared if they've thought about their own experiences in this area.

I grew up in a generation for whom coming out as something other than heterosexual was a significant life event. For many of us, it was traumatic and fraught with anxiety, but ultimately transformative in a positive way. For my heterosexual friends, coming out often seemed pretty effortless—so much so that they barely registered it. For many young people today, no matter what their sexual orientation, coming out is more as it was for my heterosexual friends than as it was for me. That isn't to say that some young people—of all sexual orientations—don't still have a difficult coming-out experience, but as societal attitudes toward nonheterosexuals become more accepting and as nonheterosexual orientations are more apparent in mainstream culture, the process of coming out is changing for everyone.

Coming out is a two-step process. We come out to ourselves first and then to others. At some point, we become aware of our sexual and romantic attractions and realize that they are directed (oriented) toward a particular gender or genders. We internalize that realization, integrate it into our conception of ourselves, and then, at some point and in some way, make that piece of ourselves known to others. It is the interplay between our own feelings and actions and the perceptions and reactions of those around us that shapes our coming-out experiences. This is different from simply assuming one's sexual orientation. Because we live in a largely heteronormative society, heterosexuality is assumed. We might even say people are presumed heterosexual until proved otherwise. It is, however, the self-recognition and self-definition of our romantic and sexual attractions that makes a coming-out experience.

Coming Out to Yourself

As young children, we experience romantic and sexual feelings for other people before we understand those concepts or have language for those feelings. The best example I can give is drawn from my own experience. See if it resonates with you. When I was a little boy of five or six, I knew I felt somehow "different." It wasn't anything I could put my finger on. It was just a general sense that I wasn't like other kids. What I *did* know was, it had something to do with Donny Osmond. Donny Osmond and his brothers (the Osmonds) were a very popular musical group back in the late 1960s and early 1970s. They were constantly featured on all of the variety shows that dominated afternoon and prime-time television in those days. When I watched

Donny Osmond, who was about seven years older than I was, my stomach felt funny—as though it had butterflies in it. I really liked looking at him, and when the song was over and he disappeared from the TV screen, I felt kind of sad. There weren't any genital feelings associated with watching Donny Osmond, and I certainly didn't know anything about sex or sexual feelings, but I *really* liked looking at him. It wasn't that I wanted to be like him or was jealous of his talent or anything else I could figure out at that age. It was just that looking at him somehow made me happy. I didn't see other boys on TV who liked looking at Donny the way I did; I mostly saw girls screaming and cheering at him. I also figured out pretty quickly that talking about my liking to look at Donny Osmond was not a good idea. Adults went silent; my boy friends told me that only girls liked looking at Donny Osmond; my girl friends totally got what I was saying but that was confusing and unsettling.

Now, what if I *had been* a little girl instead of a little boy? First of all, I'd have seen lots of other girls on TV screaming at Donny Osmond and cheering while he sang—and I'd also have seen lots of examples of girls looking at boys the way I liked to look at Donny. If I'd told adults that I liked looking at Donny Osmond, they'd probably have asked me if I liked him or even teased me about wanting to marry him someday. They'd have contextualized and normalized my feeling as the way girls often feel about a talented or attractive boy. My friends would also have normalized what I was feeling. Other girls would have shared stories about their feelings, which would have sounded similar to mine. I would have felt understood by my same-gender friends in this shared experience. And the boys might even have wanted to convince me to feel about *them* the way I felt about Donny.

Because I was a savvy little kid (as many of us who discover our difference early are), I knew that my feelings about Donny were my secret. I also knew that the world expected me to like girls. Enter Dawn in first grade.

Dawn was a very nice girl with long brown hair, and I decided I should like her. She didn't give me any of the tingly feelings that Donny Osmond did, but that didn't matter. I told Dawn I liked her and we began our first-grade love affair. One day, after saving up 25 cents, I went to the expensive gumball machine (not the nickel or dime ones) and bought Dawn a ring with a huge emerald in it.

The next day I went into the school yard, went up to Dawn, got down on one knee, pulled out the ring, and asked her to marry me. She said yes and we ran to tell one of our teachers the good news. Sister Miriam Dorothy, one of the many Catholic nuns who dominated my early education, looked down at us as we excitedly told her we were engaged and she said, "Well, that's just wonderful!" Some of our classmates teased us for being a couple, but I felt so cool!

So, what happened to Dawn? She moved away the summer between first and second grade and I never saw her again. My students often quip, "You better watch out, Mr. V, if she shows up with that ring, what are you going to do?!" I laugh and say, "I'd introduce her to my husband and tell her she can keep the ring."

These are both examples of early coming-out experiences, but they play out in very different ways. For parents who want to be more inclusive of their child's blossoming sexual orientation, think about the feedback loop you're creating with them. Are you encouraging them to talk about their feelings in whatever way they are manifesting? Are you sending them messages that sexual orientation is healthy when it's an honest expression of who we are, and that forcing ourselves to fit into a predetermined box is unhealthy? Do our kids get messages from us that normalize their feelings or ones that tell them to keep quiet about their feelings? Those early experiences create the basis for how our kids will handle other coming-out experiences in the future.

It's never too late to change the way we talk about sexual orientation with our kids. But first, it might be useful to spend some time thinking about your *own* coming-out experience. Here are a few questions I use in class to help my students get in touch with their own, individual coming-out experiences. Think about them in terms of your own life and the life of your child.

At this point in your adult life, you know what sexual and romantic attraction feel like, so try to recall your earliest experience of those feelings. Who was the first person (or one of the first people) you remember having a crush on? What was the earliest feeling or experience of puppy love you can remember? What did it feel like? Try to differentiate between events that were not attached to sexual or romantic feelings and events during which you actually *felt* attraction of some kind. You probably didn't know they were sexual or romantic feelings then. It may have felt "tingly," or "special," or like having butterflies in your stomach. Do you remember telling someone (your parents, your friends) about those special feelings you were having? How did they react? How did their reaction make you feel?

Another useful question to think about is who were your early models of sexual orientation (not gender)? What television shows, stories, magazines, and movies helped you to understand or contextualize your sexual and romantic feelings? There were probably tons of examples of heterosexual people and couples, but what about examples of people who weren't heterosexual? How were they portrayed? How did people react to them? What lessons did you take from that?

Having a personal experience or example to draw on will make it much easier to talk to your kids about sexual orientation in general and about *their* sexual orientation in particular. The fact is, whether we recognize it or not, we are *already* part of the feedback loop that is giving our kids information about their sexual orientation. Now we can be more deliberate about participating in that process, and more deliberate in communicating values about sexual orientation to the young people in our lives.

Coming Out to Others

Think about the last time you were chatting with an acquaintance or a person you recently met. Maybe you met up with a neighbor for coffee, or stopped to talk to the mother of one of your kid's friends at soccer practice. Over the course of your conversation, did you mention anything about a romantic or sexual attraction you had for another person? I'm not talking about a deep, intimate conversation, here—maybe you mentioned something about your spouse or sweetheart, or talked about a celebrity or sports star you find attractive.

Guess what? That was a coming-out experience.

Coming out to others isn't a one-time event. It's a lifelong process. Every time we meet someone who doesn't know us, we reveal information about ourselves to them both implicitly and explicitly. One of the things we reveal is our sexual orientation. Again, consider the difference between assuming a sexual orientation and presenting or confirming it in some way. Every day we meet people who will make all kinds of assumptions about us. They might assume we're wealthy or middle-class, educated or ignorant, liberal or conservative. They will also, most likely, assume our sexual orientation. That assumption will likely be implied or mentioned in conversation at some point, and we may confirm or correct it. *That* is coming out.

I talk to my seniors about experiences like this because many of them will soon be leaving for college, where they'll meet a whole new crop of people. What will they assume about their new friends' and classmates' sexual orientation? How might they talk about their sexual orientation when they are forming new relationships? If incorrect assumptions were made about their sexual orientation, how would they go about addressing that? If they have a nonheterosexual roommate or friend who comes out to them, how can they help to make that experience a positive one for the other person?

Sometimes coming out to the people we know best can be even harder than coming out to a stranger. The more important our relationship is with a person, the more care we may take in revealing aspects of ourselves to them, especially if we think it will go against their expectations of us. For instance, if parents make it clear that they assume their children are heterosexual, it can be very difficult for their child to come out with his or her sexual orientation if it's different from what's expected. Parents who talk with their children about the joy of falling in love with a sweetheart (leaving gender out of the picture, or being explicit that the gender of the person isn't an issue) make it much easier for their children to share their sexual orientation honestly once they discover it themselves. If a parent, employer, teacher, or another authority figure assumes your sexual orientation—or worse, makes it clear that they consider only one sexual orientation valid (and it isn't the one you have)—coming out can not only be emotionally risky, but may also have social, financial, and even physical ramifications.

Some people ask me, "Is it really necessary to come out to other people?" They often go on to say, "It's private information. Is it really anyone else's business other than the person I'm sleeping with or in love with?" It's a valid question, but it doesn't take into account the full impact of sexual orientation in our lives. Sexual orientation isn't just a "category" of our lives—it influences who we are and what we do, every day.

So if you tell me that "sexual orientation is private," here is my response: see if you can spend an entire day going about your normal routine without making *any* reference to your sexual orientation. No talking about your sweetheart or mate, no gossip about who you think is cute or not, no references to your past or future relationships. When people actually take on this challenge, most find that it's pretty tough to make it for more than a few hours without slipping up. That's because our sexual orientation isn't just about our most intimate moments that happen behind closed doors. Like gender, sexual orientation is a lens we use continually to interpret the world and our place in it. It influences what we say, how we say it, what we do, and how we do it. I'm not just a gay man in the bedroom. I'm a gay man in the classroom, the supermarket, my house of worship, on social media, and everywhere else. I don't walk into the supermarket and expect someone to come over the loudspeaker and announce, "Gay man shopping in aisle three," nor do I introduce myself to my students as a gay teacher, but we reference our sexual orientation implicitly or explicitly constantly. We can't hide our sexual orientation and be a whole, healthy person. That's why it is so important to help your child feel comfortable talking about his or her orientation openly with you. Those simple or not-so-simple conversations make an enormous contribution to the development of their healthy sexuality.

Sexual Orientation Prejudice

As I reentered my ninth-grade classroom, having stepped out to grab my fifth or sixth cup of coffee that day, I heard a phrase that's actually pretty uncommon in my school.

One boy groaned to his buddy, "That history test was so gay!"

I looked over at the boy who had just spoken, smiled, and said, "Congratulations!" He answered with a "Huh?"

"You must have aced the history test! Great job!" I said.

"No," he stammered. "It was so hard, like *unfair* hard!"

"Oh, but I heard you say it was so gay. Didn't you say that?"

"Yeah," he said, looking even more puzzled.

"And that means it was great, right? Even awesome, huh? So, congratulations! When I hear someone say, 'That's so gay,' I always assume they're celebrating something."

A lot of the kids in the room were just staring at me, some blankly, some confused; a few were smiling.

"No, Mr. V!" an overeager and somewhat awkward young man piped up. "When you say, 'That's so gay,' it means something was, you know, like, really bad."

"But that doesn't make any sense," I said, taking a sip of coffee. "Being gay is awesome. So is being straight, or bisexual, or whatever. Why would anyone use a sexual orientation as a negative?" Then I asked them to take out their homework and class got under way.

Each of us has our own values about sexual orientation, and those values can vary widely. We live in a society whose values about sexual orientation are complex and evolving, but whose values about individual liberty are clear. Each individual has the right to live life unencumbered by prejudice and discrimination. Sexual orientation bias, like all discrimination, exists in both overt and insidious ways. One of the core values in my class, and my life, is that sexuality education is a form of social justice education. Therefore I work with my students to recognize and combat prejudice and discrimination based on any aspect of sexuality, including sexual orientation. So when I heard "That's so gay," I knew the student was using it as a negative; that's the typical way the phrase is used in our society. But rather than lecture the young man or the class, I chose to give them something to think about, a way to reframe the idea. A thought-provoking comment, especially when it provokes a little mental puzzle, can go a lot further than a stern lecture. In my own value system—and I should also make clear the value system of the school where I teach—there is no hierarchy of sexual orientation. They're all awesome, so using any of them to signify a negative is not OK.

Let me take a moment to be clear about what I mean by "sexual orientation prejudice." I use that as an umbrella term to encompass several different kinds of prejudice and discrimination—many of which your kids may already be familiar with, either from personal experience or through a friend.

Sexism is prejudice or discrimination based on gender identity or expression. When gender expectations (boys do this/girls do that) are so rigidly enforced that people feel that they can't behave in ways that feel natural to them, that's sexism. Anytime we force a person to change the way he or she lives, works, looks, or behaves solely because of gender assumptions or expectations, we are discriminating against that person.

Heterosexism is the belief that everyone is or should be heterosexual, and the conscious or unconscious exclusion of nonheterosexual people from one's reality. In its most extreme, heterosexism denies that other sexual orientations even exist or denies that any sexual orientation other than heterosexuality is valid. In less extreme forms, it may mean classifying nonheterosexuals as inferior to heterosexuals. The most common cases of heterosexism occur when people ignore or fail to consider the possibility that nonheterosexual people are a part of their daily life.

Heterosexism can be insidious. It may not be in-your-face offensive, but over time, it erodes the status of nonheterosexuals. The next time you're in a card store, look through the anniversary cards. How many of them could be used by people in same-gender relationships? Here's another example that usually blows people's minds: Think about why bathrooms and locker rooms are divided by gender. At least one of the reasons for grouping in this way is the assumption that girls can go to the bathroom and change around each other because they aren't sexually attracted to each other. Can you see how heterosexism makes nonheterosexual people essentially invisible?

So when your child tells you about a new friend, you might ask, "What do their parents do?" rather than "What do their mom and dad do?" When prom time rolls around and kids are getting ready for the "big ask," keep your language inclusive: "Did Kathy get asked to prom? I hope she's going with someone nice." When you're filling out one of the hundreds of pieces of paper your child brings home from school, notice whether it asks for "mother's/father's" signature or "parent's/guardian's" signature. If the language the school is using isn't inclusive, why not send an e-mail with a helpful suggestion on how to change that for the better?

Homophobia, biphobia, and transphobia all have similar definitions: the fear or hatred of lesbian or gay people (homophobia), the fear or hatred of bisexual people (biphobia), and the fear or hatred of transgender people (transphobia), as well as the fear or hatred of being *perceived as* having any of these sexual orientations.

Homophobia, biphobia, and transphobia are increasingly displayed in acts of violence against nonheterosexuals. This violence can include verbal, physical, emotional, or social attacks. It may also include deliberately spreading false information, which can lead people to commit acts of violence against nonheterosexuals. Homophobia, biphobia, and transphobia result in thousands of deaths each year. They are also some of the main causes of bullying in schools. If your child is being teased with taunts of being gay, or if a bully chooses a slur to disparage the way a child is dressed, we have to do more than simply stop those comments from happening. We have to help our kids see the injustice in them.

Homophobia, biphobia, and transphobia can be expressed in lots of ways besides bullying. When we withhold or curtail affectionate words or gestures from our same-gender friends because we don't want to give the "wrong" impression, that's homophobia. When we deny that bisexuality is a real sexual orientation, dismiss it as "just a phase," or assume that bisexual people are the same as lesbian and gay people, that's biphobia. As the transgender community has become more visible in recent years, there has been a sharp increase in incidences of transphobia. Each year on November 20, the Trans Day of Remembrance honors trans individuals who have been killed due to transphobic violence. Of course, the transgender experience is not only about violence and suffering. There have also been a flurry of beautiful children's books published in recent years highlighting trans characters and their experiences.

Sexual orientation prejudice can be found in every community, even the most accepting and open ones. It begins with the failure to recognize that there are far more sexual orientations in our community than we imagine. Individuals in our community, family, school, house, or place of worship may not come out because of the sexual orientation prejudice they've seen exhibited by members of the community, even their own friends.

Eliminating Sexual Orientation Prejudice

Prejudice is born of ignorance, assumption, and fear. It's OK for you or your child to ask people about their sexual orientation in an honest attempt to get to know them—just be sure not to interrogate or judge once you hear their answer. Once your kids understand more about sexual orientation, they might have questions about the people you already know. If they ask you about one of your friends who is nonheterosexual, be honest and, if possible, provide an opportunity for that person to speak with your son or daughter directly. If it's a family member, it may require a little bit more sensitivity, but again, it's important to be honest with your child and show that there are good, loving people around him or her who are of a different sexual orientation. And the thing that seems to have the greatest impact on reducing sexual orientation prejudice is having a personal connection. When we really know someone as a whole person, as a complete individual, it's hard to discriminate.

When talking to your children (or anyone, for that matter), the language you use makes a big statement about your attitude on sexual orientation. Make it clear that you respect and acknowledge diversity by using inclusive language. If you know someone who is in a heterosexual relationship, it's fine to talk about the boyfriend or girlfriend, but if you don't know, you might want to use *partner* or *sweetheart* or another inclusive word.

Another way we convey our true feelings about sexual orientation is through humor. Jokes can often reveal our prejudices as much as our wit, and those offhand comments that fly out of our mouths can do a lot of damage. Remember that your kids are watching and listening to each of those comments, and making assumptions and judgments about what is right and wrong based on your words. Before you make a "harmless joke," think about how you would feel if you overheard your child making a similar joke. Would you be embarrassed? If so, it's probably not that funny. And when others make a barbed remark, speak up. Every time we let a comment, joke, or insult slide by, we're contributing to sexual orientation prejudice.

In the end, curbing discrimination requires us all to speak up and step up when necessary. There is so much emphasis on educating young people about bullying these days, but sexual orientation prejudice is just as pressing a problem on today's school campuses. By setting a positive example, help empower your kids to be positive influences in their school and in the world around them.

Question Box

Q: What percentage of America is openly homosexual?

A: The traditional answer is that somewhere between 1 percent and 10 percent of the population is gay or lesbian. I know that sounds like a huge range, but we really don't have any accurate way to count people according to their sexual orientation.

The other thing to think about with this question is exactly what it means to be openly homosexual. People can be "out" to various degrees. Some gay and lesbian people tell their friends about their sexual orientation but not their family; others tell people close to them but not people at their jobs or people who know them only slightly; still others are totally open about their sexual orientation. All of these things can count as being "openly homosexual," although some people think only the third example listed fits the definition.

Q: How do two guys dance together?

A: I like this question. It's not one I've gotten before! If you're talking about slow-dancing, in which one person leads, there are a couple of ways for same-sex couples to figure that out. Sometimes the taller person leads; sometimes the person who's the better dancer leads; sometimes they take turns leading. Sometimes couples talk about who's leading before they start to dance, other times they just go out onto the dance floor and do what feels natural. Now when it comes to fast dancing (as they used to call it when I was a kid), you just go out onto the dance floor and shake what the good Lord gave ya—same as any couple.

Q: How do two girls have sex?

A: This is one of the most common questions I get asked as a sexuality educator. Let's just look at the question for a second and see what it tells us—and then I promise I'll answer it.

So many people associate the idea of "having sex" with vaginal intercourse, for which, of course, you need a penis. Yet two women having sex together don't have a penis, do they? Nope, they don't. Then some people say, "Oh, they must use some kind of sex toy or artificial penis!" Yet the research shows that only a small minority of women who have sex with women use a sex toy or penis substitute as part of their sexual activity. Then people really get confused! This question reveals to us how much we value the penis and how closely we adhere to the baseball model. If we were more able to think about sex according to the pizza model, we'd remember that the penis is only one part of a whole body that can be used to give and receive sexual pleasure. Give the poor penis a break! There's a lot more there to work with!

OK, so to answer the question, sex between women includes all the kissing, caressing, and stimulating that sex between a man and a woman or a man and a man does. The vulva is often stimulated with the hand or the mouth, and since that's where the clitoris is, the potential for orgasm is greatly increased by this kind of stimulation. Some women do stimulate the vagina as well, using fingers or a sex toy, but as noted above, not the majority of women.

The best sexual activity doesn't come from a manual or a

list of instructions. It comes from knowing your body, knowing your partner's body, and communicating about what brings both people pleasure. That's what we all should do when we engage in sexual activity.

Q: What could it mean if you have only extreme sexual attractions to one gender but extreme emotional and (only slight) sexual attractions to the other?

A: This is a great question because it recognizes that we have different kinds of attractions.

• Sexual Attraction: Whom we feel turned on by and want to have sexual activity with. This is a body response; it's about seeking and giving sexual pleasure.

• Emotional Attraction (also called Intimacy): Whom we feel closely connected to and whom we want to know more fully and deeply. This isn't about sexual activity necessarily; it's about sharing trust, communication, and those intangible aspects of ourselves.

• Romantic Attraction: Whom we want to form a loving relationship with. Romantic attraction is more than just wanting to hook up with somebody. Some see it as a combination of sexual attraction and emotional attraction. It's about wanting to know someone deeply and share sexual pleasure with that person.

In terms of your question, I'm afraid you're the only person who can determine what your various attractions "mean" for you.

It's not uncommon that we feel strong sexual attraction to one gender and strong emotional attachment to the other. In fact, it's not uncommon for people to have stronger emotional connections with the gender(s) they're *not* sexually attracted to, because all that confusing anxiety that can come with sexual activity is set aside and you can just focus on the other aspects of each other. A healthy romantic relationship is successful when two people can develop their emotional attractions for each other while also maintaining and acting on their sexual attractions for each other. This isn't always easy, but most people in good romantic relationships will say it's worth it!

....

CHAPTER 7

OK, So I Have a Body. How Do I Like It and What Do I Do with It?

Of all the topics we cover in the Sexuality and Society class, none must be handled with more care than body image. Talking about the anatomy and physiology of genitals during our sex and gender unit is a walk in the park for kids compared with exploring how they feel about their bodies and how that relates to how they use their bodies.

The reason for this isn't all that hard to understand. Most people, especially adolescents, don't feel very good about their bodies. How can they when we live in a society that tells them every day that they're not thin enough, in shape enough, buff enough, pretty enough, or normal enough? And age doesn't insulate adults from these messages either; how many of us would cringe if we were asked to explore our own feelings about our bodies?

I always give plenty of advance warning when we're moving into the body-image unit. Some kids need to put on their best defensive armor for those classes. Once in a while, kids simply won't show up for a class, not because they're being melodramatic but because it's just too hard for them to have to think about their bodies in a group of their peers.

The activity we do at the start of this unit can be found at the end of this chapter. It's a simple list of body parts; the work comes in when I ask my students to rate their level of satisfaction with each part of their own bodies. As with all in-class activities, students may decide how much or how little of the activity they want to do. Their emotional safety and well-being are far more important to me than filling out a handout.

In processing the activity, some themes emerge that carry through the rest of the unit. First, students note that what makes a body part satisfying can be different for different parts. Sometimes it's about appearance: "I'm dissatisfied with my feet because I think they look weird." They also quickly realize that this level of satisfaction or dissatisfaction is highly correlated to how they perceive how *other people* view those parts: "I rated my eyes highly satisfying because people often tell me they're pretty." Other times body parts are rated in terms of the way they function: "I rated my uterus low because I get really bad menstrual cramps." Or: "I don't like my ankles because they're weak and I sprain them a lot."

Second, I've rarely had a student rate every part of his or her body as satisfying or highly satisfying. Everyone feels some level of body dissatisfaction and anxiety, although there is a great variety of ways this can be expressed. Getting to the reason *why* this is so takes more time to explore and understand, but it's important to establish right away that no one in class is alone in feeling awkward or less than satisfied with some part of his or her body.

Third, students begin to see that body image is influenced by culture, ethnicity, class, and other nonbiological factors, and that these influences may be positive or negative.

At the end of the activity, I hand out blank index cards and invite the students to write down the part of their body that they're *most* satisfied with. They don't put their names on the cards. I fill out a card too. Then I collect the cards, and we hear a litany of positive comments about our bodies. With that little shot of love in the room, we're ready to move into the topic in a deeper way.

Body Image: The Bad News

The tricky thing about body image is that it's not really about how we look. It's all about how we *think* we look. The definition of body image is the mental image we have of our physical appearance. It's crucial that young people understand this definition, because improving body image is all about changing how we think about our bodies; it's not about actually changing our bodies.

Poor body image is an epidemic in this country, and this is especially true among young people. Body dissatisfaction, dieting, and overexercising to lose weight or change body appearance (rather than to be healthy) begin in grammar school. More and more adolescents are undergoing cosmetic surgery before their bodies are even fully developed. Disordered eating continues to be a substantial problem in that population. The book *I'm, Like, SO Fat!* reports that more than half of teenage girls and nearly one third of teenage boys use unhealthy weight-control behaviors, such as skipping meals, fasting, smoking cigarettes, vomiting, and taking laxatives.*

The media and our consumer culture are the main culprits in the body dissatisfaction epidemic. We are constantly presented with images of seemingly perfect bodies and told that if we buy the right diet plan, pills, cosmetics, workout plans, or surgical procedures, we can have that perfect body as well. Body dissatisfaction is big business; people are making millions of dollars from reinforcing our body insecurities. This cycle can be broken only if we expose the lies about those images of perfect bodies in the first place.

I think it's helpful for young people to understand that the photos presented to them everywhere—in magazines, on billboards, in movie theaters—aren't real. Each image represents one moment frozen in time, and hundreds of photos are taken to find the one frame—the one millisecond—that looks the best. Then that photo is digitally altered to bring it to even more impossible standards of beauty. There is an amazing YouTube video I always show to my classes titled "Dove: Evolution." It's less than two minutes long, but it has a huge impact on the kids. Produced by the Dove Real Beauty campaign, it uses time-lapse photography to show a model from the moment she walks into the studio to the moment her image appears on a billboard. In between those two moments are hours of makeup and hair styling, hundreds

....

* Dianne Neumark-Sztainer, *I'm, Like, SO Fat!* (New York: Guilford Press, 2005): 5.

of photos taken with special lighting and filtering, and then the chosen image is digitally modified. The woman's eyes are enlarged, her neck is lengthened, her shoulders are narrowed, her skin is airbrushed. The final image that appears on the billboard is stunning, but it bears little relation to the actual woman who walked into the studio at the start of the clip, who is perfectly lovely in her own right. I follow this up with other videos that show photos of the students' favorite celebrities and musicians before and after they have been digitally altered. There are many different versions of these videos also available on YouTube. Film and video representations are no different. They use all manner of makeup, lighting, and filters on cameras to enhance and alter people's appearance.

My students are stunned when they see these videos. No one has ever made it so clear to them that the images they see in magazines and on TV are *based* on real people, but have been significantly changed. It's also important to point out to them that the women who are used in fashion ads are not anywhere near average to begin with. The CDC reports that the average American woman over twenty years old is about five feet four inches tall and weighs an average of 170 pounds.* The average fashion model is around six feet tall and weighs between 100 and 130 pounds.† A young woman in my class who works in a popular store selling women's clothing

....

* *Anthropometric Reference Data for Children and Adults: United States, 2015–2018*, Centers for Disease Control and Prevention, https://stacks.cdc.gov/view/cdc/100478.

† Lauren Effron, "Fashion Models: By the Numbers," ABC News, September 19, 2011, https://abcnews.go.com/blogs/lifestyle/2011/09/fashion-models-by-the-numbers.

said the mannequins they typically use in her store are a size 0. (The average American woman wears a size 14.) If those mannequins were real women, they'd have less than 10 percent body fat. Before my students start to think that's a good thing, I remind them that a woman needs 13 to 17 percent body fat to maintain a menstrual period. Their reactions to all this information range from betrayal to anger to deep sadness. It is the rare young person who feels vindicated by this news, and the ones who do typically came into the classroom with a healthy body image.

Lest we think media images don't have any real impact on kids, 47 percent of girls in fifth through twelfth grades reported wanting to lose weight because of the pictures they see in magazines.[*] And research published in the *International Journal of Eating Disorders* reveals that 42 percent of girls in first through third grades want to be thinner than they are.[†] In addition, studies have shown that people who read magazines frequently are three times more likely to exercise for the goal of weight loss rather than health, and were also three times more likely to have unrealistic body expectations.[‡]

....

[*] Alison E. Field et al., "Exposure to the Mass Media and Weight Concerns Among Girls," *Pediatrics* 103, no. 3 (Mar. 1999).

[†] M. Elizabeth Collins, "Body Figure and Preferences Among Pre-adolescent Children," *International Journal of Eating Disorders* 10, no. 2 (Mar. 1991): 199–208.

[‡] Alison E. Field et al., "Exposure to the Mass Media and Weight Concerns Among Girls," *Pediatrics* 103, no. 3 (Mar. 1999); Marian M. Morry and Sandra L. Staska, "Magazine Exposure: Internalization, Self-Objectification, Eating Attitudes, and Body Satisfaction in Male and Female University Students," *Canadian Journal of Behavioural Science* 33, no. 4 (Oct. 2001): 269–79, doi: 10.1037 /h0087148.

Another exercise we do in my class is to examine children's toys to see what kinds of body expectations are being represented to very young children. There have been many studies about how Barbie's body is not comparable to any human being's, yet few parents tell their children that Barbie could exist only in a fantasy world. In fact, if a woman did have Barbie's actual body proportions, her neck would not be strong enough to allow her to lift her head, and her ankles and feet would not be strong enough to allow her to walk upright—she would need to crawl around on her hands and feet (and Barbie's very narrow wrists would make that difficult as well).

But it's not just toys marketed to girls that provide problematic body images. The musculature of most male action figures today if put onto a real man would be grotesque. Harrison Pope's study of male action figures shows that in 1964, G.I. Joe had a thirty-two-inch waist and twelve-inch biceps.* The 1991 version of G.I. Joe had a twenty-nine-inch waist and sixteen-inch biceps. In 1995 G.I. Joe Extreme was introduced, with biceps that would be twenty-seven inches around in a human being, larger than those of any bodybuilder ever known. I show the students the Superman action figure I played with in the 1970s and compare it with the Superman action figures available today. My Man of Steel is positively puny when compared with the contemporary Man of Steroids. When I wanted to dress up as Superman, my costume came with an "S" to sew onto a shirt and a red fabric cape. Today, they come with molded plastic muscles, and some even inflate to give a boy a seemingly massive (and grossly distorted) body.

....

* Harrison G. Pope Jr. et al., "Evolving Ideals of Male Body Image as Seen Through Action Toys," *International Journal of Eating Disorders* 26 (1999): 65–72.

Body Image: The Better News

Building a better body image is possible once we understand that it's about changing our thinking rather than actually changing our bodies. Remember, what we think we look like is not what other people see when they look at us. There are three important ideas I've found that help with improving my students' body images.

The first is that human bodies come in three basic types. Ectomorphs are naturally tall and skinny. They have a hard time putting on weight or muscle mass, although they easily show the muscle definition they have. Most female fashion models are ectomorphs, and our societal idea of female beauty favors ectomorphs. Mesomorphs have bodies that are of average build. They can gain or lose weight and can put on or lose muscle mass without significant difficulty. Many male fashion models, especially those with highly sculpted, muscular bodies, are mesomorphs, and our societal idea of male beauty starts with this body type. Endomorphs are naturally rounder in shape. They have a hard time losing weight and while they can gain muscle mass, they don't typically achieve the "chiseled" look our society favors. Endomorphs are unlikely to show six-pack abs; even though they may have core strength, they usually have excess body fat covering the muscle.

The most important thing to understand about the three basic body types is that you can't alter your body's essential underpinnings—you are born with a body type, and all you can do is make it the healthiest and best body for you. In class I use cars as a comparison. Cars are built with distinctly different frames—compacts, sedans, SUVs, etc. You can put all kinds of fancy options onto an SUV, but it's still an SUV. This was not a lesson I learned when I was a young person, but I wish I had.

I'm an endomorph, just like my dad. I'm on the short side, broad chested, and generally heavier than average. My brother, a classic ectomorph, is naturally skinny. As a kid I was always uncomfortable with my body. I wanted to be tall, skinny, and blond rather than the short, dark-haired, fleshy guy I was. When I would complain about my body, I was told that all I had to do was exercise and I could have whatever kind of body I wanted. That was a lie. I exercised as a kid and a young adult, but whenever I looked in the mirror, I was still that short, broad, dark-haired kid. Given that my ethnic background is entirely Italian, it's exactly what I should be, but no one ever helped me see that and appreciate it. For too long I gave up on exercise and any thought of having a body I could love, all because I never learned to love and accept my body type. By the time I learned that lesson in my adulthood, I was so deep in body shame that it's a constant struggle for me to love the body I have. I share this story with my students because if they can assimilate the message about loving their base model early enough, they, unlike me, can avoid chasing an impossible dream.

The second idea is to be clear about what it means to be fit and healthy versus what it means to follow a societal standard of beauty. Fit doesn't have a specific weight requirement, musculature, or body hair distribution. Understanding what's fit for one's own particular body means knowing that, for the vast majority of us, it isn't the body the media is trying to sell us. In addition to this, I believe it's helpful to think about how, in so many ways, we "live in the middle," as I like to say. No matter what physical attribute, talent, or quality we can name, there will most likely be someone better than us and someone not as good as us. As I tell the kids, "There is only one most beautiful person on the planet. There is only one best dancer." Then I point to myself and say, "There is only one sexiest person on the planet," and am greeted by cheers, laughter, and sometimes puzzled looks.

When it comes to our bodies, there will always be people who were dealt a better genetic hand, aesthetically or functionally, and there will always be people who would love to have a body like ours. This idea really helps to level the playing field for kids. No matter where you are on some imaginary scale of body beauty, the vast majority of people are in the middle of some pack or another. This is also why it's so important for kids to have friends with all different kinds of body types. Kids who hang around only with people who look like them are much more likely to be competitive with each other about beauty or body type. Yes, competition can be healthy, and wanting to better ourselves is admirable, but we can't use impossible standards as our goal to achieve our best, healthiest selves.

The third idea I present when we talk about improving body image is to ask each student to make a list of all people who matter most to them—friends, family, sweethearts, coaches, whoever. After they've generated the list, I ask them to review it and circle all the people who are on that list specifically because of the way they look. Rarely are any names circled. I also ask them to pay attention to the adults they know and look at whom those adults choose as sweethearts. Real couples in real relationships don't pick each other solely because of their physical features. I ask them to think about the couple they know who are most in love with each other—not a celebrity couple but people they actually know in their lives. Sometimes they think of their grandparents, or an older sibling, or even their parents. How many of those people have bodies like those they see in magazines and on TV? Not many.

A Word About Body Hair

In discussing body image with young people today, the issue of body hair is one that has to be addressed. Cultural preferences for hairy versus smooth bodies wax and wane (pun intended). In the 1970s, a hairy chest was the preferred look for men, and pubic hair was considered perfectly normal and even attractive for both men and women. Today we live in a culture that doesn't seem to like any amount of body hair. Removing all hair below the neck is the trend, whether by shaving, waxing, or any number of other painful procedures.

These days, kids start trimming or removing their pubic and body hair as soon as it comes in. They will argue it's purely for aesthetic reasons, which raises the question: why is body hair unattractive? But I think there's a lot more going on than that.

Kids always ask if it's OK to shave or trim their pubic hair and body hair. They want a quick answer; I want them to explore the why behind the question. I have a quip about body hair that always makes the kids laugh, and then think. I say, "Humans are mammals, and all mammals have hair." And then add, "If you didn't have hair, you'd be a lizard." As I want all of my students to be in charge of their own bodies, I never tell them they can't trim or remove their body hair. There's nothing fundamentally unhealthy about doing that. I just want to really make them think about *why* they're doing it and ask themselves if they're OK with that answer.

It's important to think about the reasons why we have body hair and pubic hair, and also the timing of *when* we get the majority of our body and pubic hair. Hair that grows in during puberty is a sign of sexual maturity. It's a way to differentiate reproductively capable adults from those who are immature and not capable of reproduction. So what signal is sent when postpubescent people choose to groom themselves in the style of prepubescent people? I ask my students all the time, "If you're all in such a hurry to grow up, how come you want your bodies to look like you're still eight years old?" I have a theory about this. It's not scientifically tested, but I've gathered lots of anecdotal evidence in support of it from high school students, college kids, and adult audiences. I wonder if shaving pubic hair and body hair is a way of subconsciously trying to escape the adult responsibilities involved in sexual activity and sexual relationships. I think there's an "if I look like a little kid, then I can act like a little kid" mentality that pervades our culture, and I don't think it's healthy at all. Of course, this is just an idea. There are lots of other reasons why kids today might shave or trim their body hair. It could simply be about wanting to appear youthful and not connected to sexuality at all. Or perhaps girls want to look younger because they think boys like younger girls. And as with any adolescent behavior, kids may start to groom their pubic hair simply because their friends are doing it and because they are in a locker room with teammates who are shaving. Again, the crucial question to ask (and conversation to have) is about the why.

The body-hair question brings up another important point we have to think about and talk about with young people. When a society no longer distinguishes between prepubescent and post-pubescent bodies, how does it treat actual prepubescent people and their sexuality? Starting in the late 1970s, children have become ever more sexualized in American media and culture. I graduated from eighth grade in 1978. That same year, Brooke Shields, who is a year younger than I am, starred in the movie *Pretty Baby*, playing a child prostitute. The societal uproar was enormous. How could such a young girl be cast in such a sexual role, the critics cried! Soon after, Shields starred in a series of television commercials for Calvin Klein jeans with the seductive slogan, "Nothing comes between me and my Calvins." This also prompted a public outcry. Fast-forward to today, when clothes for little girls are emblazoned across the butt with words like "juicy," "sexy," and "booty call," and lots of people (including the mothers who purchase these clothes for their daughters) think it's cute. We can't pretend that blurring the lines between sexual maturity and immaturity won't have social consequences. It has profound implications for the development of healthy sexuality. Healthy sexuality for a fifth-grader isn't about being "hot" or "sexy."

One way parents can help their children develop sexually at a healthy pace is to work against the tendency to make kids appear or act older than they really are. Is what your child wearing appropriate for the chronological age and the development of his or her body? It's OK to tell our children that some things are not appropriate for them because they're simply too young for that. A great example of this comes up every Halloween, as costumes for women and girls become skimpier and sexier. You can't just dress up as a witch or a nurse anymore; it has to be a "naughty nurse" or a "sexy witch." Even costumes that have nothing to do with gender, like an outfit in the form of a candy bar, have become sexualized for women. A guy who wants to be a Hershey's Kiss gets to wear a big, baggy, shiny triangle, while a woman gets a silver bra, silver go-go pants, and a Hershey's sash to tie around her bare waist. We look at ads for Halloween costumes every year in my class, and the kids are always grossed out by the blatant sexism. Are we questioning things like kindergarten proms where five-year-olds are expected to pair up, dress up, and go to a dance together? (I'm not kidding—this happens!) Whether your child is invited to a coed sleepover, a costume theme party, or a school dance, I think it is always important to ask the question, "Is this age appropriate for my child's physical, emotional, intellectual, and moral development?"

Body Image and Sexual Activity: The Connection

The psychiatrist and author Anthony Storr once said, "We cannot escape our physical natures; and a proper pride in oneself as a human being is rooted in the body through which love is given and taken."

There is no doubt that body image has an impact on the way we approach sexual activity and behave during it. A good body image is correlated with increased sexual pleasure and satisfaction, while a poor body image is correlated with the reverse. The reason is pretty simple: the most satisfying sexual experiences happen when the people involved are fully present in the moment and fully understand and appreciate their bodies. When we are worried about our bodies during sex, it's much harder to be present enough to enjoy ourselves. A poor body image may also lead to avoidance of all sexual relationships or sexual activity. And a poor body image may prompt some people, especially young people, to participate in sexual activities they don't really want to engage in because they think that's all someone who looks like them deserves or can get.

For teenagers, their changing bodies are an endless source of fascination. Most of the fun that teenagers poke at their bodies comes from insecurity. They know that their bodies are supposed to feel good to them at the same time that they're mystified and often horrified by all of the changes taking place in them. They generally feel pretty out of control when it comes to their bodies.

Many, if not all, of the questions my students ask about their bodies and sex are anxiety fueled: *How do they know if they're ready to have sex? Is it normal to masturbate more than once a day? Does the first time always hurt?* They're less interested in hearing me talk about the play-by-play of what happens during sex, which is good because, as I often remind them, it's not a how-to course. They're all ears when I begin to deconstruct the emotions, misconceptions, and sometimes shame that accompanies having a body and using it for sexual purposes. They want to know if it's OK to be so simultaneously scared and interested. And above all, "is it normal to . . ." (fill in the blank). I've had kids ask if it's normal to feel awkward when making out or having sex with someone (yes!) and normal to have to be talked into sex by your partner (no!).

Ultimately, they're saying, "OK, Mr. V. I have this body. So what do I do with it?"

Building a Relationship with Your "Junk"— Kids' Views of Genitals

You may be familiar with one of the slang words used today for genitals: *junk*. I really dislike that term, which is often used among high schoolers. In my opinion, we'd be a much more sexually healthy society if we had an open and complete understanding of our bodies and were honest about the fact that our genitals are far from "junk."

Talking about genitals with my students is tricky. I don't want them to think of their genitals as the most important parts of their bodies when it comes to sexual activity, but I need to talk about genitals in order to make that point.

"It's important that you know what your genitals look like and feel like, and what kind of stimulation is pleasurable and painful for them," I'll tell my students. If you're going to take your body into a sexual situation with somebody else, you've got to be an expert on your own body first. It's going to be difficult to give and receive pleasure without knowledge of your body.

If there's any part of a young male body that he thinks he knows everything about and yet is endlessly curious about, it's the penis. By the time they reach puberty, most males have already established a complex relationship with their penises. How can they not? Penises are pretty obvious; males look at and touch them multiple times a day for both sexual and nonsexual purposes. Males receive explicit and implicit messages about their penises all their lives. The penis gets called things like "manhood," "tool," "spear," "snake," and any number of other aggressive names. A male begins to hear that power and success are connected to the penis. Our society is pretty accepting of talking about penises in serious and not-so-serious ways.

Don't get me wrong, penises are great, and I'm glad when males can become familiar with their genitals and feel good about them. But the preoccupation can sometimes be taken too far. I love announcing to my classes, "Penises aren't light sabers! They don't ejaculate the cure for cancer! They're just penises." The kids roar with laughter, but they also get the point. Guys can easily go from feeling penis pride to having penis arrogance. It stops being an organ for sexual, reproductive, and intimate uses and pretty easily gets thought of as a weapon of power and dominance. On the flip side, those whose penises are smaller than average (or at least they perceive them to be smaller) may suffer needlessly from feelings of inadequacy. We need to address all these ideas when we talk about bodies and sexual activity.

Even my students, whom I consider sophisticated and savvy, get hung up on penis size. They believe all of the myths: *A bigger penis is a better penis. Every other guy has a giant penis except for me. A bigger penis feels better during sex.* If I had a nickel for every time the question, "What's the average penis size?" was placed into my Question Box over the years, I'd be a very wealthy man. The message about penis size, whether from the media, the schoolyard, or porn, is that they come in three sizes: huge, gigantic, and so big they drag on the floor. That's obviously not reality. So I look forward to dropping this piece of data, which tends to open their eyes.

The vast majority of fully grown males will have an erect penis that measures somewhere between 5 and 7 inches, with the largest concentration between 5.5 and 6.5 inches. That's it. Yes, some have penises that are larger than average and some have penises that are smaller than average, but remember, we live in the middle. The size of the penis when it's flaccid (not erect) is no indication of the size it will be when erect. As the saying goes, "Some are show-ers and some are grow-ers." I always add, "Ultimately, smaller than average, average size, or larger than average, penis size is just a number. It doesn't matter at all. Love what you have and your life will be much better."

Because our society is hung up on penis size, they also assume that a bigger penis means more sexual pleasure and satisfaction for them and their partners. Again, this is not true. It's important to understand that penis size is not the only determining factor in sexual pleasure. Believing that the mere presence of a penis ensures sexual satisfaction makes a person a lousy lover.

When it comes to the subject of female genitals, society is much quieter. There is not much encouragement to know one's vulva or be proud of it. Most people have seen an image of a penis by the time they're in high school, even if just in an art museum. But you don't typically see images of vulvas as regularly—they remain hidden, and many females internalize this, thinking that a vulva is something no one wants to look at. The kids are shocked when I show them pictures of a variety of vulvas to illustrate just how much they vary. Unlike penises, which tend to look pretty similar, vulvas come in an amazing array of shapes, colors, and sizes. The labia can be symmetric or asymmetric, the inner labia can be longer than the outer labia, the clitoris varies in size from person to person. The range of normal for a vulva is expansive and wonderful. Yet rather than appreciate the unique beauty and variety of vulvas, there's a trend today to make vulvas as "pretty" as possible. Some even go to the extreme of undergoing plastic surgery on their labia to make their vulvas look "better."

Boys are typically mystified by how little girls know about their vulvas. "What do you mean you don't know what you look like?" a boy will always challenge the girls.

The girls will squirm a bit in their chairs before one bravely pipes up: "You can't just look at it—it's kinda hard to see!"

"But an empowered, healthy person *should* know what their vulva looks like," I'll tell the class. "I'm serious. Take a few minutes, go somewhere private, get a mirror, and take a good look." Besides looking, getting to know the sensitivity of one's vulva is important. What parts respond best to touch? What's too much sensation? There's no shame in a teenager examining themselves and learning about their bodies. In fact, it's an important part of coming of age. If a teenager doesn't know their body, they can grow to be ashamed of it and not feel in control when it comes to guiding sexual activity. We get so many messages in pop culture about vaginas being dirty or gross, but I want my female students to know that their genitals are actually amazing, beautiful, and pleasurable. I want to try to increase vulva pride! My students know I'm gay and they often assume I'm grossed out by vulvas. I may not be sexually attracted to them, but I think they're amazing. It's important that we change the conversation about female bodies, so they feel more confident about them, whether they're in a sexual situation or not. I talk about them with awe and enthusiasm, and getting to know and understand the natural beauty of vulvas has made many young people in my classes feel better about having one. Some kids ask me, "Mr. V, are you *sure* you're gay?" I'm sure.

Students are especially enlightened when I report that Go Ask Alice, Columbia University's premier website for sexual health information, says that the average vagina is three to four inches deep when not sexually stimulated and five to seven inches deep when stimulated. In other words, it's made to accommodate an average-size penis. "Vaginas aren't endless passages to Narnia," I'll joke. "If someone has a longer-than-average penis, it's going to bump the cervix, which actually really hurts girls. Those boys have to be especially sensitive partners."

Answering Questions About Masturbation

Years ago I taught in an all-boys high school. Frequently the young men would come to me with questions or concerns about sexuality. One day a young man made an appointment to see me about "something really serious." I brought to the forefront of my mind all the things this usually meant: a pregnancy or STD scare, possibly a coming-out story, questions of whether a relationship is ready for sex, or even, God forbid, reports of abuse. I steeled myself for a tough conversation.

He was visibly upset when he came to see me. He wouldn't

look me in the eye, and he fidgeted constantly. I told him that I was open to hearing whatever he wanted to tell me and that I wasn't going to judge him. I also gave him the caveat every teacher needs to give a student who comes to talk: "You need to know up front that if what you tell me makes me think you are in danger of harming yourself or someone else, I can't keep that information confidential."

"No," he said, still looking down at his fidgeting hands. "It's nothing like that. It's just . . . Well, I don't think I'm normal."

"OK," I said. "Is there something you're doing that makes you think you're not normal?"

"That's just it!" he said, raising his voice and then instantly lowering it again. "I'm not doing anything. I mean, I'm not . . ." and his voice trailed off.

"I can see this is hard for you," I said, "and I'd really like to help if I can, but I'm not exactly sure what you're talking about."

He mumbled a string of words so quickly and softly that I could make out only the word *off*. "One more time?" I asked.

"I don't jerk off," he said. Saying that opened the floodgates for him. He told me he had tried masturbating a few times but didn't like it, and he didn't feel that he needed to do it. He wasn't in a relationship and wasn't sexually active in any other way. He just didn't like masturbating. It wasn't that he thought masturbating was wrong or dirty. It just wasn't for him. The last thing he said before he stopped talking was, "I know I'm pretty screwed up, right?"

We talked for a while longer, and I assured him that he was perfectly normal. Masturbation isn't a requirement of adolescence or of any other phase of life. Some people like it, some people don't. We talked about how guys tend to assume that every other guy masturbates, and how guys freely talk about masturbation. But some of this is just talk. If adolescent guys masturbated as much as they say they do, they'd never have time for anything else. I said, "It's not like all the other guys are cutting class to go masturbate. I mean, they're there in class with you, right?" That made him giggle.

....

If you're a parent of a teenager, you can safely assume that your child has at least experimented with masturbation. Really, it's not a question of do or don't; it's a matter of what role masturbation can play in helping to develop healthy sexuality.

While it is true that not everyone does, or has to, masturbate, masturbating can be an important way for young people to get to know their bodies. If teens know what feels good to them, they'll know how one day to tell someone else what they like and don't like when they're getting intimate. Not only is it pleasurable, but masturbation can also help relieve stress. Simply put, an orgasm is the release of built-up tension. When our bodies are stressed or become sexually aroused, we begin to store muscle, nerve, and vascular tension. Think of it like compressing a spring; all that energy gets stored up as the spring coils tighter and tighter. An orgasm in our body is like suddenly releasing the spring. All that stored-up energy is let loose in a rush that feels great and leaves us in a very relaxed state. An orgasm doesn't distinguish between sexual tension and tension from anxiety; it clears it all away. After studying for tests, navigating the emotional ups and downs of high school, as well as coming to terms with the changes in their bodies, teenagers need a way to release their stress. Masturbation is one way to do that. During my time at the boys' school, a photo of me in the yearbook had the caption: "Ask Mr. V about his cure for headaches." All joking aside, an orgasm can be very helpful in relieving a tension headache, and has also been shown to help reduce menstrual cramps. There's no reason in my mind why my students shouldn't know that. For parents wary of thinking about their kids masturbating, rest assured that masturbating is a safe and very normal way for teens to discover their bodies. And for those young people who don't masturbate because they don't like it, they don't want to, or it violates their value system, they need to know that they are perfectly normal as well.

A lot of myths about masturbation still exist, and some teenagers need help distinguishing truth from fiction. Few teens believe the old tales about masturbation making hair grow on your palms or ruining your eyesight, but some boys still worry that it will disrupt their athletic performance (it won't) or that they'll use up all their sperm cells (they can't), and some girls worry that masturbation will make sex with a partner less pleasurable (it won't). The big thing kids ask me is if it's possible to masturbate "too often." The frequency of masturbation among young people varies tremendously. The normal range spans from never to several times a day. The frequency also varies within a young person's life; one may go through periods of frequent masturbation and then may decline or stop for other periods. This is not a place to worry about what's normal, because the range of normal is so wide.

Conventional wisdom says that boys masturbate more frequently than girls, but that idea is affected by our societal views about penises and vulvas, as we saw earlier in the chapter. Society also allows boys to talk about masturbation much more freely than girls. The difference I've witnessed in this is that boys will talk about masturbation at the cafeteria table no matter who else is sitting there. Girls might talk about it with their close friends and usually only in private settings. There are boys who masturbate at home in the shower, in the bathroom at school, or in their bedrooms. Sometimes boys will masturbate together (which does not necessarily have anything to do with their sexual orientation). Many boys masturbate before bed because it helps them fall asleep. It's true that a young person can get so turned on during school—remember, their hormones are raging, so it doesn't take much—that they might take a quick trip to a private place so as to refocus on lessons.

I tell my students that the important question isn't whether they're masturbating too little or too much, but rather, what's the place of masturbation in the larger context of their lives? If masturbation becomes an obsessive or intrusive part of your life, that's a problem. If you'd consistently rather stay home and masturbate than go out with your friends, then that's a problem. If you make your genitals sore by masturbating too roughly or too much, but you keep doing it anyway, that's a problem. For some people, masturbation is against their personal, family, or religious value system, and doing it makes them feel guilty. To act consistently against one's values and suffer guilt as a result is a problem.

There is one conversation about masturbation that parents really do need to have with their sons. Every year a practice called autoerotic asphyxiation tragically takes the lives of young people, almost always young men. This is the act of restricting one's airflow during masturbation, usually by fastening a belt or rope around the neck. Cutting off the oxygen to the brain heightens the feeling of an orgasm, but this is an extremely dangerous practice. People can and do inadvertently strangle themselves. Every adolescent needs to know that it is never OK to restrict the airway in any way while masturbating.

Girls also masturbate, of course, and while my female students don't deny it in my class, they're much less comfortable talking about it than their male counterparts. It's important for girls to understand that masturbation is as normal for them as it is for the boys. And beyond normalizing this experience for girls, I also think we can share the empowering message that their sexual pleasure does not depend on a penis. The clitoris and labia are the main areas of stimulation in female masturbation; these are also the primary sites for stimulation that results in orgasm for women. According to *The Hite Report: A Nationwide Study of Female Sexuality*, a famous 1976 study, upward of 70 percent of women say they don't regularly orgasm through vaginal intercourse alone.[*] This is eye-opening for the boys who, as teenagers and sometimes into their adult years, often assume that rough sex is what feels most pleasurable to girls.

I wonder: if we help young people understand their bodies and what brings them pleasure, do you think we might actually see a decrease in intercourse among young people? Despite what is depicted in the media and pornography, intercourse isn't necessarily the best or only option for sexual pleasure and orgasm.

It's perfectly OK to give your kids permission to explore and

....

* Shere Hite, *The Hite Report: A Nationwide Study of Female Sexuality* (New York: Seven Stories Press, 2004): 512.

touch their bodies, genitals included, so that each can understand their body and its response to touch. You don't even have to use the word *masturbation*, if it makes you feel uncomfortable. Let's be clear: I'm not suggesting you say to your child: "Go to your room, fantasize, and pleasure yourself." That would be way outside most parents' and kids' comfort zones. And certainly I, as a sexuality educator, would never say that to a kid. But do give them facts. You might say, "You'll hear all kinds of things about masturbation, but it doesn't do any physical, mental, or emotional harm to a person, and for lots of people it's a normal part of life." You might also review your family rules about privacy, assuring your teenagers that you respect their right to have time to themselves for whatever purpose. It takes nothing more than a simple statement, like "I'll always knock before I come into your room if the door is closed, and it's OK to tell me that you need privacy." At that point, your child may run screaming from the room—or may surprise you and ask a question about masturbation. If you don't panic and shudder in embarrassment, chances are, they won't either. And if you talk to them about their genitals the way that you would, say, about keeping your heart healthy or your skin clear, with the wisdom of experience, it will make the conversation less awkward for you as well.

I frequently remind kids how important it is to try to love your body, especially if you expect anyone else to love it, and that one way to love it is to know it. "If you're ashamed of your body or think your body is gross, what is the gift you're giving to someone else?"

"Am I Ready to Have Sex?" and Other Questions Kids Ask About Their First Time

Most people are incredibly nervous the first time they have any kind of sexual activity with another person. Just reading that sentence may prompt you to recall your first time and how you felt. Losing your virginity, however that's defined, is generally an experience met with some anxiety and nerves. Kids wonder: *Am I ready? Will it hurt? Is it normal to be so scared? How will I know if I'm doing it right?* I end up answering those same questions each year for a new crop of kids, which goes to show how universal these fears are.

In my opinion, the best way to start a conversation about losing one's virginity is to figure out exactly what virginity means and what value a young person attaches to that term. Virginity has traditionally meant not having engaged in penile-vaginal intercourse. Some people also include not having had penile-anal intercourse. Few, if any, teens today include not having had oral sex in their definition of virginity. There has traditionally been a double standard to loss of virginity: heterosexual boys are expected to lose it while heterosexual girls are expected to preserve it. Some people still consider virginity until marriage an important value for everyone; some consider it important for women but not for men; and some no longer value retaining virginity until marriage. It's important for parents to talk with their teenagers about what value virginity has for them and what place it holds in their family values. It's also important to avoid legalistic definitions of virginity that are full of loopholes or that are not inclusive of lesbian, gay, bisexual, and transgender people. My own definition of virginity is "not being involved with another person's body with the purpose of achieving sexual pleasure." So in my book, having oral or anal sexual contact counts as losing one's virginity—but that's just my personal opinion. I tell this definition to my students but also make it clear that what's most important is that *they* know what *they* mean by virginity, and that they're sure they know the definition of virginity of any potential sexual partners.

While few adolescents want to know anything about their parents' sex lives today, it can be very helpful for parents to share lessons they learned from their early sexual experiences. Of course, not every parent is comfortable doing this, but for those who are, opening up to your kids about your first time can be incredibly helpful to them. Parents are often afraid that if they share details of their own adolescent sexual experience, somehow it will translate into a permission slip to go have sex. Quite honestly, kids aren't seeking your permission. You're not opening the door; you're guiding them through their innate sexual curiosity. Try one of these conversation starters: "One thing I wish I'd known my first time is . . ." or "My first time was great because . . ." or "My first time was awful because . . ." When you tell the story with the gift of perspective, you're able to pass along some very powerful lessons to your kids. Kids learn well through storytelling. Here are some examples:

I felt rushed to do it the first time because all of my friends had done it, but I didn't really like the person I did it with. I think it would have been better if I really liked them.

One thing I wish I'd known my first time was how awkward it was going to feel. The movies make it seem like it's effortless, but it's actually kinda clumsy. It's easier if you're willing to laugh at yourself.

My first time was great because we were so in love with each other. We'd been dating for a while and we'd talked about the fact that we were both ready.

My first time was awful because my parents walked in on us—and it was the most embarrassing moment of my life.

Look for the lesson in your early sexual experiences, and pass that along to your kids. Play up the part of your story that you want them to learn from most, and don't be afraid to share vulnerable moments. Be prepared for follow-up questions and let them know that it's OK to ask them.

"How Will I Know If I'm Ready?"

Kids love to ask this tricky question, and the answer "If you aren't sure, then don't do it" is limited in its usefulness, because it doesn't help kids figure out what it means to be sure. It's also important to acknowledge how personal the answer to that question is; there's no one right answer for everyone. A 2019 CDC study found that about 20 percent of males and females reported having had sexual intercourse before they were fifteen. That number increases steadily to around 50 percent by age seventeen and 70 percent by age twenty. Overall the average age of first intercourse has declined over the past twenty years. It's now roughly eighteen years old. Accurate statistics for the frequency of same-sex sexual activity among young people are difficult to find, but rates of about 10 percent for females and 3 to 5 percent for males are often cited.* It's also important to note that data is neither destiny nor instruction; they're just numbers, which may apply in a particular person's case or not. For me, the most important aspect of being ready is the ability to think beyond oneself. I always ask kids if they're able to talk to their potential partners about having sex— that's one big indicator of being ready, in my book. My rule for sexual activity—for kids, adults, senior citizens, whomever—is, "If you can't look your partner in the eye and talk about it, you shouldn't be doing it with them." I know that's not the way most of society operates, but remember, our society isn't very healthy when it comes to sex. Another important question is, "Are you as concerned with the pleasure of your potential partner as you are with your own?" And another: "Are you as aware of and concerned about the potential consequences for your partner as you are of your own?" A lot of sexual activity is very selfish, and even in high school some kids just use one another for sexual pleasure. I tell my students that a healthy attitude toward sexual activity is: If I'm going to feel good, you should feel good, and if I'm getting positive consequences out of it, you should too.

....

* "CDC Releases 2019 Youth Risk Behavior Survey Results," Centers for Disease Control and Prevention, last updated August 20, 2020, https://www.cdc.gov/healthyyouth/data/yrbs/feature/index.htm.

"What If I'm Nervous?"

I'd suggest telling adolescents it's natural to be nervous, that it would be strange if they *weren't* nervous, because they're thinking about doing something they've never done before. You might also help them distinguish between being nervous and being afraid. If they're truly feeling afraid, then it's time to go back and reconsider the plan. Fear can be a sign that something's missing in the equation: Maybe the couple hasn't adequately discussed contraception or safer sex? Maybe the time or place or person isn't right? Being nervous is a natural reaction to approaching something we haven't done before. It doesn't mean we don't want to do it. Think about riding a roller coaster. If you're feeling nervous that it might be scary, you'll probably stay in line. If you actually fear for your safety, you're likely to bail. Being nervous is not necessarily a bad thing. It can make us more attentive and more deliberate—things that can be really helpful the first time a couple is sexual together.

I warn my students against using alcohol or drugs to curb nervousness before becoming sexually active. "If you can't do it completely sober," I impress upon my students, "then I don't think you should do it at all!" They don't like hearing this, but *I've* heard too many snippets of what happened at the latest high school party, and it's clear that kids are not always making sexual decisions with a clear head. Another of my absolute "must haves" for healthy sexual activity is positive, active consent. This doesn't just mean the absence of a no; it means the presence of a clear, active yes. When alcohol or other substances are involved, positive active consent becomes unlikely and perhaps impossible for both partners. I try hard to press the point that going to a party entails making a deliberate either/or choice: either the substances or the sexual activity but never both. My students *really* don't like hearing that, but I keep saying it.

"Does It Hurt the First Time?" "Will I Bleed?"

I never mislead kids to think that their first time will be like the movies—it never is—and I also don't make them think it will be awful. The truth, as always, is somewhere in the middle. Yes, there can be pain the first time a couple has penetrative sex. It's a lot less likely if the couple goes slowly and pays attention to each other's words and actions. This also means it's essential to speak up if something hurts. If the partner being penetrated is feeling relaxed and ready emotionally, they will be less tense. If one is anxious or afraid, one's body is going to be tense, muscles are going to be more clenched, and that can make it hurt more. Time, communication, honesty, and plenty of lubrication are the keys to reducing pain during first sexual activity. Sometimes there is a little bleeding during first vaginal intercourse, especially if the hymen has been ruptured, or during anal intercourse, but the couple may not even notice. Penetrating too quickly or forcefully or not using enough lubrication can make intercourse painful and make bleeding more possible.

"What About My Hymen?"

This is a common question from girls. The hymen is a thin, natural skin membrane that may cover part of the vaginal opening. The first thing to establish is that not all women have hymens. Some are born without them, which is completely normal. A hymen can't be used as proof of virginity because some women never had one to begin with. In eras when women were not expected to be physically active and before tampons were used during menstruation, women's hymens often did break during their first experience of penetrative vaginal sex. When a hymen breaks in this way there can be a moment of sharp pain and some bleeding. Today, most girls born with hymens have broken them long before their first experience of intercourse. Anything from riding a bicycle to doing a cartwheel to exercising to inserting a tampon can cause a hymen to break. Most girls probably aren't even aware of it when it happens this way. It is important for a female to know whether or not she has a hymen when she is considering having penetrative vaginal sex for the first time. If a hymen is present and a woman doesn't want it to break during first intercourse, she can go to her gynecologist, who can easily and painlessly remove it or perforate it so it's not a factor during sexual activity.

"How Far Is Too Far?"

This is where I go back to my pizza model I discussed at the beginning of the book. If a teenager's goal is satisfaction, then not everyone has to have intercourse, or even an orgasm, for an encounter to be satisfying. Some people are completely happy with cuddling and kissing. Sometimes you just want to feel close to someone for a little while. The only way to know if something is far enough or too far is for there to be clear communication. I prefer verbal communication to nonverbal cues, which can be misinterpreted. Again, honesty is essential. Each partner is responsible for assessing his or her own level of comfort and desire and requesting that same information from the other person. My students often say they don't want to hurt their partners' feelings when something doesn't feel good. But what they don't know is that their partners would love feedback. Feedback during intimate moments is a good thing. Here's another moment when I drum into my students' brains the idea that "only positive, active consent counts as consent." Saying nothing is not consent. Doing nothing is not consent. The best way to keep a sexual experience from going too far is to continually check in with each other and assess. Simple questions like, "Is this OK?" "Do you want to . . . ?" and "Can I . . . ?" can make a world of difference. Nonverbal communication can work, but it's more open to misinterpretation, and clarity is key in consent. If an intimate moment does go further than intended, it's essential to think about why and to learn from it. Did you find it difficult to speak your mind? Did you push your partner or yourself to do something because you felt pressure to do so from friends? "There's no rule book about this stuff," I'll tell my kids. "The two of you are writing the rule book as the experience unfolds, especially the first time you're sexually active with each other. It's all a part of figuring out what feels right and what doesn't, and that is empowering for both of you."

In the classroom, I often go back to a silly analogy to help my students see what I mean. I tell them to picture themselves snuggling with their sweetheart when suddenly they begin to lick your eye. Profusely. It doesn't feel remotely good. It's actually pretty gross. You're thinking, *OMG! Licking my eye? Ewwww!* "How long would you let that continue," I ask, "and how would you make it stop?"

Someone will always offer, "I'd just say, 'Stop licking my eye! I don't like that.'"

"Exactly!" I say, and we all laugh at the thought of the scenario. "That's a great example of a clear statement that says 'too far.'" The command "Stop licking my eye!" sometimes becomes a refrain in class after that. Both the kids and I use it to put a stop to something that's become annoying or unpleasant. "Mr. V, stop licking our eyes!" someone will shout when I drift off into a story I've told a hundred times before. "Enough with the eye licking!" I'll call out when the students seem more interested in their cell phones than in our lesson.

Pregnancy and More: What Can Happen When You Have Sex?

Most of my students are pretty savvy about how someone gets pregnant. Many of my female students are on some form of birth control, either because they've asked their parents for it or because their parents have suggested it to them. According to the Guttmacher Institute's research, 77 percent of females and 91 percent of males used contraceptives the first time they had vaginal intercourse.[*] There are many reliable forms of contraception besides the birth control pill, and they don't require daily attention. If you're not someone who will remember or think it's

....

[*] "Adolescent Sexual and Reproductive Health in the United States," Guttmacher Institute, September 2019, https://www.guttmacher.org/fact-sheet/american-teens-sexual-and-reproductive-health.

important to take a pill every morning, then another form of birth control is needed. The birth control patch needs to be changed only once a week; the vaginal ring, once every three weeks. One Depo-Provera injection is needed every three months; an IUD or birth control implanted in the upper arm) can work for years. It's essential to talk with your child and their doctor about birth control, even if they're not yet sexually active. Birth control pills may also be used for other health purposes—such as regulating periods or lessening the severity of menstrual cramps.

Each method of birth control has its benefits and drawbacks, so it's important to consider the full range of options and not just opt for the same method you or your cousin or friend is using. Pregnancy is one of those spots where there *is* a rule book. If you consistently use reliable contraception, you can feel confident that you won't get pregnant. Decisions about birth control can be made independently of the decision to have intercourse, which is why it's helpful for parents to talk to their children about birth control options *before* they're also trying to make a decision about engaging in intercourse. That way, the birth control decision is based on what's best for the young person, their body, and their life—and not the fastest and easiest option so that the sex can start. Of course, in a long-term relationship, partners should discuss birth control options together.

Beyond pregnancy, there are other discussions to have about protective behaviors during sexual activity. Sexually healthy people know how to protect their bodies from STDs. Make sure your kids are clear that no form of hormonal birth control will protect against sexually transmitted diseases like chlamydia, HPV, herpes, or any others on the standard STD list. I don't think it's useful to get out a chart of STDs with lots of gory pictures and scare your child silly about what they could catch. From years of experience, I can tell you it goes in one ear and out the other. What's most helpful for teenagers is to tell them what they should look out for on their own bodies. If you know your body and you've looked at it enough, you'll know when something out of the ordinary appears on it, like a sore, a lesion, or an unfamiliar discharge. It's also important to know which STDs are bacterial (and therefore curable), which are viral (and therefore incurable), which are transmittable through oral sex or skin-to-skin contact, and which STDs condoms may not be effective in preventing. Being knowledgeable about Gardasil, the vaccine that prevents the strains of HPV (human papillomavirus) associated with an increased risk of cervical cancer, genital warts, anal cancer, and vaginal cancer, is also essential, although decisions about receiving this vaccine should always be discussed with a health care provider.

"When you're getting sexual with someone, keep the lights on—at least at the start," I'll tell them. "It's important to see your partner's body, both to really appreciate it and to make a quick visual inspection. You should make sure they're as sexually healthy as you are." In other words, you'll be able to make an informed choice about whether or not you want to be physical with someone who may have signs or symptoms that can signal an STD. I suggest to my students that anyone who is sexually active should be tested once per year, especially if they're sexually active with more than one person.

My students always laugh when I tell them, "The first thing my parents taught me how to do was worry, and over the years,

I've gotten really good at it." Sometimes I wish I could be more carefree, like my students. I love how invulnerable they think they are, even from things like STDs. I hate for you to take that feeling away from them by scaring them senseless about diseases or other negative consequences. Still, a healthy dose of reality is in order. A perfect line to deliver to your kids is: "I don't want you to be scared of having sex—I just want you to be smart." Kids know what you mean when you say you want them to be smart. You're telling them you want them to make an informed decision. You're giving them the information and the value context to make a decision, and you're putting the ball in their court. Kids appreciate that.

"Keep the lights on," I'll holler out to my students as they walk out the door at the end of the period. That's my way of keeping them smart.

Red-Faced: When You Walk In On Your Kids

You and your sweetheart get home from dinner with friends. You go upstairs to check on your sixteen-year-old. You knock, open their door, and find your child masturbating. The two of you lock eyes in terror. Red-faced and flustered, you turn around, slam the door, and run downstairs. *How will you ever look your child in the eyes again?*

What's the right way to handle a scenario like this? The above example is not that far off. I tell parents that the best way to handle walking in on their kids masturbating is to say, "Oops, I'm sorry," close the door, and walk out. You don't want to freak out—the conversation can happen later. Freaking out shames children into thinking that they're doing something wrong. They're not—they're doing something private. I don't think that that moment is the time for a conversation about masturbation, although when you do have that talk, make sure you let your children know that it's a normal part of their developing sexuality. Instead, it would be good to talk about issues of privacy. "I'm sorry," you might tell your child. "I should have waited for you to say it was OK before I opened the door."

Walking in on your child having sex with someone else is a whole different story, and there are a couple of appropriate responses. First of all, if your child is in bed with someone you don't know, you have every right to ask them to stop right then and there and get dressed—and you can wait there while it happens.

If your child tells you that it's his or her sweetheart but you didn't know they were dating or you never met the person, you might say, "Well, this isn't how I expected to meet. I'd like to get to know you, but put on some clothes first." If your child is in a relationship you know about with a person you've met, then the rules may change, especially if you've established that it's OK to be sexual together in your home. If so, maybe you can say, "Oops, I'm sorry," and leave, as if you walked in on your child masturbating. If you haven't established any rules about sexual activity in your home or the behavior you come upon is violating those rules, then that's what needs to be addressed. You can have the conversation with the couple or with your child alone. It's important that both child and sweetheart know your rules about sexual activity in the home. Is there a family rule that says that when you're with your sweetheart, you're not alone in the bedroom? Once you establish a rule and they break it, then the conversation isn't about the sexual activity. It's about breaking the family rule.

....

Question Box

Q: How do disabled people have sex?

A: One of the first things to note about this question is that it all depends on the definition of sex. If we're using a very limited "baseball" definition of sex as vaginal intercourse, then those whose disability leaves them with no sensation in their genitals wouldn't be able to have sex. If, however, we use a more pizza-based definition of sex that isn't solely focused on genitals or vaginal intercourse, then people can have satisfying sexual experiences in all kinds of ways, so people's disabilities or differences may not affect their sexual lives at all.

The question is also difficult to answer because people can have so many kinds of physical differences. People who are paralyzed below the waist have little or no feeling in their genitals but often find that another part of their body is especially sensitive to sexual stimulation and may receive sexual pleasure in that way. People with other kinds of physical disabilities that don't involve paralysis or loss of feeling may experience no difference in their sexual activity when compared with someone who isn't disabled. People with intellectual disabilities and differences have whatever sexual activity is appropriate to their level of intellectual development.

The important thing to remember is that people with physical or mental differences are fully sexual human beings and enjoy pleasure, intimacy, love, and sex just like people who don't have disabilities.

Q: Can girls really have orgasms?

A: Absolutely!! Orgasms are a biological event that both human and nonhuman animals, male, female, and intersex can experience. An orgasm is a sudden release of muscle and nerve tension that produces a very pleasurable feeling throughout the whole body, usually starting from the genitals and radiating out to the rest of the body. When people are not having orgasms, it's likely that they're not receiving the kind of stimulation their bodies need to get to the point of orgasm or that they're nervous, anxious, tense, or otherwise not able to relax into the experience and let their bodies do what they want to do. There is a myth that it is harder for a woman to achieve orgasm than it is for a man. This isn't actually true. What is true is that knowledge of how to bring a man sexual pleasure that might lead to an orgasm is much more widespread than knowledge of how to bring a woman pleasure that might lead to an orgasm. Here we see that sexism again; we're expected to know about men's bodies but not about women's.

Q: Are you a semi-virgin if you had oral sex but not intercourse?

A: The question I have in response to your question is what's the value of being a "semi-virgin"? As we discussed in our classes, there is no one definition for the term *virgin*. It can mean many different things to many different people. We should start by asking the question: Why is the label "virgin" important? What benefits and drawbacks come with that label? Are the benefits and drawbacks the same for men and women? We might see sexism again here, as virginity is often seen as a desirable quality in women but not in men. Why is that? Is that fair?

According to my definition of virginity (never having interacted with another person's body in order to give and receive sexual pleasure), having oral sex means a person is not a virgin. What does your definition of virginity tell you, and why does that answer matter?

Q: What's the average duration of sex?

A: This is a great question but one that's hard to answer. Often this question focuses only on the length of time vaginal intercourse takes, from when the penis is inserted into the vagina until the male ejaculates. (Notice how that definition is both heterosexist and sexist. It doesn't include gay and lesbian couples and the endpoint is defined only by the male ejaculating; it says nothing about whether the woman has achieved orgasm or not. Here's a great example of the baseball model at work!)

If we're using the pizza model instead of the baseball model, this question becomes unimportant. Sexual activity should last until both partners feel satisfied. Each act of sexual activity wouldn't need to be compared with the next or the last one. Why worry about how long or short the activity is if both people feel satisfied at the end of it? Remember, it's not a competition.

BODY RATING EXERCISE

··

PART I—INDIVIDUAL RATINGS

Directions: Listed below are various parts of your body. Your task is to rate your satisfaction with each individual body part. You are not comparing body parts here, but are looking at each one individually and determining your satisfaction with it. Use the following scale:

1 = very dissatisfied   2 = dissatisfied   3 = neutral
4 = satisfied   5 = very satisfied

Rating	Body Part	Rating	Body Part
	neck		uterus / prostate
	hair (on your head)		thighs
	hands		eyes
	fingers		teeth
	vagina		waist
	calves		nose
	knees		stomach
	buttocks / butt		abdominals
	feet		vulva / penis and scrotum
	breasts / chest		mouth
	arms		ears
	shoulders		back

Rating	Body Part	Rating	Body Part
	tongue		nipples
	face (entire)		toes
	skin		body hair
	ovaries / testes		pubic hair
	belly button		lips
	hips		wrists
	eyebrows		earlobes
	height		weight
	other (specify)		other (specify)

PART II—TOP/BOTTOM FIVE

Directions: Go back to the list in part I. Write the five body parts that received the highest scores or with which you are most satisfied and the five body parts that received the lowest scores or with which you are least satisfied in the spaces below:

MOST SATISFIED (TOP FIVE):

1)

2)

3)

4)

5)

LEAST SATISFIED (BOTTOM FIVE):

1)

2)

3)

4)

5)

PART III—REFLECTION QUESTIONS:

Directions: After completing parts I and II, reflect on the questions below.

1) Were there body parts left off of the lists that you found yourself thinking about? Which ones? Would they get positive or negative ratings?

2) Were there body parts that you realized you don't think about much? Why don't you think about them?

3) What makes a body part one that gets your attention versus one that gets ignored by you?

4) What feelings were you aware of when you were completing this exercise? Did those feelings surprise you? Why or why not?

5) Overall, what did this exercise suggest about your own body image? Does that please you? Why or why not?

....

#iloveyou: Teens, Sex, and Technology

My father and his family were big storytellers. When he got together with his siblings and cousins, they didn't talk about politics or religion or current events; they talked about the past. They told stories from their childhood. They reminisced about people who had died. They relived events from years past as if they had happened just last night. My cousin Mary Ann would scoff at the adults sitting around the kitchen table with their coffee cups, their cigarettes ablaze. She referred to their nostalgic musings as "taking the Buick out of the garage for a ride." Bear with me for a moment as I head for the garage and take my own Buick out for a brief spin.

When I was in third grade, my father called my brother and me to the dining room table for "an important talk." We, of course, thought we were in trouble, but we weren't. My father was sitting in his usual seat looking serious and somewhat worried. He said he wanted to show us something that we should know about but *never* touch. He took a small something down from the top shelf of the corner cupboard, far above where we could reach. As he sat back down, he held it with a reverence reserved for something in church. It was a pocket calculator, one that could add, subtract, multiply, and divide all by touching a few buttons. And that's all it could do, by the way—no percentages or trig functions and certainly no graphing. It performed only the most rudimentary math functions—and it was the most technologically advanced device in our house. He told us that we were never to use "it" (the calculator was referred to only as "it," as if to speak its name were to release its inner demons), especially for homework. It was an adult tool. If we used "it" to do our homework, we would never learn math properly, and that would do permanent damage to our intellectual growth. I never used "it," never even tried to, and failed my next test on subtraction anyway.

Fast-forward to today. I use a three-tone meditation chime to begin my classes each day. As I explain its use to my students on the first day of class, they look at me as though I'm some hippie guru, but it's just a simple way to focus. I tell them the first tone invites us to stop whatever we're doing. The second tone invites us to take a gentle breath and clear our mind. The third tone invites us to place our focus in this present moment, to center ourselves here and now, and to commit to being here for the class block. The whole thing takes about thirty seconds, and it's really effective when students can do it. Often, however, they're distracted by a buzzing in their pants. No, not from our more sexual conversations . . . but from a received text, tweet, or Instagram DM.

Our school's technology policy allows students to have their cell phones with them during the school day and to use them for academic, social, and entertainment purposes during nonclass periods. They may be used in class with teacher permission. Watching my students and their phones, it's hard to know sometimes who is in charge. Their responses to each buzz, beep, or ping are Pavlovian. It calls, they respond—even when they know they shouldn't (like during the chime time at the start of class). This situation isn't unique to students. Oftentimes the people who are texting them are their parents, even though the school asks them not to do this. The parents of my students are just as technology dependent as their kids are. I'm the last generation who grew up without these tools. I'm not saying that was better, just different.

I am not immune to the draw of this technology either. I was a late adopter, but once I got my first smartphone there was no going back. And it's not just about keeping up with social media. My cell phone is my clock (remember wristwatches—so retro!) and helps me monitor my diabetes by giving me updates on my blood sugar levels. It's been an amazing means to keep in touch with former students and friends from long ago. It's the last thing I look at in the evening and the first thing I look at when I wake—and that worries me.

In the "olden" days of teaching, like the late 1980s, when I started, young teachers sought to perfect their "teacher eyes." When well trained, they could spot a cheat sheet, a passed note, an attempt to put gum under the desk, or a sly foot signal (point left for true and right for false) in an instant. Today it's all about spotting the hidden cell phone in use. This year I had a student who mastered the art of balancing the phone in the crook of his elbow and texting as if he were scratching his arm. I've spotted cell phones inside hoods, up sleeves, under desks, and even hidden in wads of tissues. And it's not that kids are engaging in academic dishonesty with their phones. There are no tests in my sexuality class, so there's never a need to cheat. It's just that they can't imagine being unplugged for the forty minutes of class. They *have* to know what's happening and there's always someone who wants to tell them something *right now*! Even the most interesting class activity will take a backseat to an incoming text message.

Cell phone use in school has also created another unexpected consequence—I find it degrades the community connections, especially between students and teachers. When students have access to their phones during the school day, a whole other level of community and conversation exists completely separate from what's happening on the face-to-face level. There are times in my class when it's obvious something is up; the kids are reacting to something, or energized about something, or angry about something but I have no idea what it is. Now, I'm not someone who wants to know everything that's going on in my students' lives; establishing appropriate and healthy boundaries is part of my job. Before cell phones there was certainly student drama, but it wasn't quite as immediate or ongoing as it is now. Even my most captivating lesson can't compete with a flurry of messages about the latest gossip or rumor that's taken off. I can, and do, collect phones at the start of class with my ninth-graders, which helps a little bit but doesn't solve the problem. A classroom community can't be built on a two-tier system.

....

Like it or not, technology is changing the way that we communicate. Parents text their kids throughout the school day, while students snap each other from their smartphones, even when they're in the same room. Instagrams announce breakups and makeups and are often annotated with hashtags—phrases used to label the online snippets so as to provide context for everyone reading. (For example, look at the difference between the same status updates with different hashtags: I Love You #wishyouknew and I Love You #forever.) Social scientists are studying the short- and long-term impacts of electronic communication on our connections to other humans. Will we, like the characters in the Pixar movie *Wall-E*, become people who rarely speak directly to each other and instead spend our days video chatting and pecking out messages in 144 characters? Probably not. Let's hope not. But electronic communication and social media are undoubtedly changing the way kids talk to one another about sex, fall in and out of love, even how they argue. And like everything we've discussed in this book, it all needs to be put into context so that we can help them think more critically and objectively about whether their behavior in the digital world aligns with their and your values in the face-to-face world.

Teens are taking multitasking to a whole new level. Multitasking today often involves talking to several people at the same time. Kids are texting at the speed of light with their sweetheart, while instant messaging with their BFF on the computer, scrolling through social media updates, and e-mailing their teacher back about a missed homework assignment. It's dizzying just how quickly they read and respond to multiple messages, and how they can seemingly take in so much information at one time and not get lost. Or maybe it just looks as though they're not getting lost? I certainly can't say for sure.

Kids today are so reliant on smartphone communication that it isn't uncommon for teenagers to begin relationships via text.

Rather than approach someone at school, they'll begin a conversation by text message: "Hey. What are you up to?" All of that time we oldsters used to spend talking on the phone, your kids spend texting. Kids ask each other their deepest thoughts over text. They complain about their soccer coach or the lousy grade they got on a biology test. They share their sexual desires, sometimes even sending provocative photos to one another. They break up via text, and say I love you for the first time. I'm sure that all adults who have teens in their lives have seen all of this firsthand.

Certainly during the COVID lockdown, we were especially fortunate to have reliable electronic communication. It kept us in touch, in school, at work, and connected to vital information about the pandemic. As we begin to return to the outside world, we are finding life changed. Working remotely isn't only possible, it's preferable for some businesses and individuals. Kids who are too sick to come to school but not sick enough to be in bed can Zoom into classes and not miss valuable instructional time. Unfortunately, this also means that snow days aren't automatically a day off anymore; they can just as easily become virtual school days. It's always a mix of good and bad.

I think using electronic communication when you have the option of face-to-face communication is problematic. Think about how much our kids, and we, miss out on. We're a species that has evolved to communicate verbally and nonverbally simultaneously. If we're not talking to someone in person, we're getting far less information. We don't see if our sweeties shift their eyes when we say we care for them, or how someone's face can help us know whether the phrase "You're too much" is meant as a compliment or a complaint. Electronic communication can be like communicating with someone who speaks a different language—a lot can get lost in translation.

It also feels to me like a shortcut, and sometimes I worry that my students choose this route to avoid the hard work of actually communicating face-to-face. My students will argue that they *are* having serious conversations via text or social media, even conversations about values, feelings, and sexual readiness. Then when they're together they can skip right to hooking up or just talk about *whatever*, since everything was discussed already via text. I have colleagues who argue that if kids have important conversations through texting, it's because they can't or won't have them face-to-face, and having them in some format is always better than not having them at all. I see that point, but I'm still uncomfortable with it. I know how teenagers fear being awkward, and I also know that healthy relationships are ones that can deal with awkwardness without avoiding it. Maybe I'm being too much of a purist here, but I want the kids I teach to push themselves to do the hard work and not settle for what's easier or more convenient or less awkward. I encourage my kids to think about why they're using text to say something so significant to their sweethearts, or to anyone. Are they taking a shortcut? Why is it difficult for them to express their feelings in person? Do they use text as a supplement to in-person communication, or do they use it as a crutch? It's also important to ask about how sincere they are in their electronic comments. When it comes to bullying, power games, or coercion, people can hide behind their devices, and that can make it hard for the recipient to know what's really going on. There's also the question of what you can "get away with." Kids can flirt with multiple parties over text and e-mail much more easily than they could in person. It's easier to deceive someone.

I'll challenge my students: "Next time you're about to text something to your sweetheart, why not call them instead? Let them hear your voice. It's OK if you sound scared or if you crack a joke to break the tension. Just say hello."

"We're not allowed to make calls with our phones during school hours!" they snap back. It's true; our school policy allows them to text or surf the Web but not actually to make calls. They're supposed to use a school phone for that.

"OK," I acquiesce. "I don't want to get into a policy debate. What I'm really interested in is this—if you had the option to either call or text your sweetheart, which would you do?"

They give me that most maddening of teenage answers: "It depends." They'll ask for clarification. "Is it a serious conversation or just, you know, something quick like a check-in?"

"Let's say it's kind of serious; not a major breakup or fight, but an important conversation."

The answer I get consistently is text for serious conversations and voice for silly stuff, the exact opposite of what my brain tells me the answer should be. But, I remind myself, I'm old, and I didn't grow up in a world that had the option of electronic communication when I was a teenager. Maybe I would have made the same choice. But the question remains, is it the *healthy* choice?

Another problem I see with relying on electronic communication is that we tend to put our best selves online—the version of ourselves that we want everyone to see, not necessarily who we really are. That increases the potential for disappointment when we do spend time with someone face-to-face. It's easy to construct a fantasy person in one's head based on clever texts and cool Instagram photos. The person in real life can't possibly compete with the one a teenager has created from building these words and images into a person. Any of us who has ever used an online dating service knows that reading someone's profile or having a short chat with them can't convey the totality of a person. What's important to realize about the way kids get to know their peers today is that oftentimes they have quite extensive and long-term electronic contact before actually meeting a friend or sweetheart in person. It's not just the initial contact that's made over text. Often the early stages of the relationship are carried out this way as well.

That long-term electronic communication can also foster a false sense of intimacy. We've all read those horrible stories of Internet predators who befriend and seduce young people by making them think no one else understands them or really knows them like *they* do. That's the most extreme case, and it's not what this chapter is about. But it shows that what looks and feels like intimacy to one person may be something entirely different to the person on the other end of the device. Here's a much more mundane example using my own circle of friends: I'm a big Facebook user and love reconnecting with people. I've had the experience of chatting with an old friend and commenting on someone's status update and feeling really close to these people, even though I may not have seen them in years or spoken to them very often. But is that intimacy I experience even real? And is it intimacy that springs from this interaction or just an echo of the intimacy I established with them earlier in our lives? Or perhaps the better question to ask: is that intimacy shared? Maybe my friends feel it, or maybe

I was a little blip in their day hardly worthy of notice. People will argue that the same thing can happen in a face-to-face interaction, but I think it'd be much easier to see that one of us was more into it than the other in that situation.

Recently out to dinner at a restaurant, I saw a family sitting at a table together. Mom was on her smartphone; Dad was on his. The two teenagers were on their phones too. No one at the table was talking. We all use our smartphones to get things done—they make everything easier. But seeing this family reminded me of the importance of knowing and living one's values. Parents will tell me that it's easier to ask their son or daughter personal questions or check in with them over text or e-mail. But that, too is a crutch. Texting and e-mail are not how you want to talk to your kids about emotions or healthy sexuality, or any kind of relationships, for that matter. If you're able to sit down with your child and talk in person about things that are bothering you, to have a conversation about values or safer sex, then you're modeling how to communicate face-to-face. If a parent is relying on text to communicate, that's a powerful message too. Sitting down and talking shows the children that the parents rely on real life to share with one another. They tune in. They put the smartphone down when it's time to talk. And they don't immediately turn to it and start texting when conversations get tough.

....

Texting and posting about relationship status is just the tip of the iceberg, though, when it comes to teens, sex, and technology. You have probably heard the term *sexting* by now, but just in case you've been spared this particular cultural phenomenon, *sexting* is the term used to describe sexual behavior in which people (often teens and young adults) send explicit text messages, photos, or short videos via text. A 2018 study published in the *Journal of the American Medical Association* (*JAMA*) reported that at least one in four teens are receiving sexually explicit texts and e-mails. At least one in seven are sending sexts. More than one in ten teens are forwarding sexts without consent, and about one in twelve teens have had sexts they've sent forwarded without their consent.*

You might ask the logical question, then: why do teens send them? The answers are complex and reveal kids' deep-seated needs to feel noticed and accepted and loved. Some teens reply with a sext because they feel it's what's expected of them. Some do so because they know it will allow a conversation, and maybe an interaction, to happen afterward. Sexting can be a gateway to starting an interaction, a hoop to jump through or something to get out of the way so the "real" communication can begin. Heterosexual young women have said that requests for a sexy photo are the first messages they get when trying to start an online conversation with a new boy.

I think it's essential for parents to talk to their kids about sexting and other cybersexual behavior—and that conversation needs to start with a discussion of *privacy*. How do your kids define privacy in a world where their everyday behaviors—what they eat, what they wear, where they go, whom they talk to—are on public display via any number of social media outlets? How

....

* Sheri Madigan, PhD, et al., "Prevalence of Multiple Forms of Sexting Behavior Among Youth: A Systematic Review and Meta-analysis," *JAMA Pediatrics*, 172, no. 4 (Apr. 2018): 327–35, https://doi.org/10.1001/jamapediatrics.2017.5314.

can they be expected to understand the difference between information that can and should be kept private and information that is meant for "sharing," after they have come of age in a digital era when virtually every bit of personal information is in the public domain? Talking about privacy with your kids means discussing family values about privacy, pointing out the long-term implications of sharing private information digitally, and allowing your kids to speak candidly about their views on privacy and what their friends and peers are doing online. You may find that your child isn't entirely comfortable with so much sharing but feels pressure to keep up socially by mirroring friends' behavior.

Another part of the online privacy conversation should focus on the impact of online sharing on your kids' future goals. Many teens are concerned about getting into their choice of college, so they're particularly shaken when they hear that college admissions officers probe social media when considering whether or not to admit a student. "If an admissions officer can see sixty-five photos of you drunk at a party," I tell them, "that's going to have an effect on their view of you." Some students have changed the name on their accounts to something other than their real name, but if I see that "Party Flo" is friends with thirty kids whom I know are seniors at the same school, it's not rocket science to figure out who Party Flo really is. Besides the fact that Big Brother is watching, safety is another issue that needs to be discussed in conversations about privacy. The potential of what kids post online to be used to harass or bully them is very real and needs to be made clear.

There's a lesson called Circles of Intimacy that was originally designed to help teach young people with developmental disabilities about establishing and maintaining physical boundaries.* The lesson uses a visual aid—a series of colored concentric circles, with one large circle on the outside and smaller and smaller circles contained within it. The innermost circle represents the student alone. It's a person's private space. Moving outward into each succeeding circle, students place the people in their lives in terms of the amount of physical contact they would share with each: who they would hug, shake hands with, wave to, or have no contact with. The activity has been adopted and adapted by many sexuality educators into a lesson about online privacy, and it may be a helpful way for you to talk about this issue with your child. Simply draw a series of concentric circles on a piece of paper. The innermost ring—the bull's-eye—represents the things a person doesn't want anyone else to know. These are the most private things in a person's life, things one doesn't share with *anyone* else. The next circle out contains information you would share only with the people you trust the most. Ask your child to think about who would be in that circle and what kind of information they would share with each of them. The people in that "most trusted" circle could range from a best friend to an aunt, a sweetheart, a teacher, etc. (When teens are being honest, parents are unlikely to be in that first circle. Don't panic, it's normal.) Ask the same two questions as you work your way to the outermost circle—who's in this circle and what information will you share with them? The last circle represents strangers. What would your child want a stranger to know? Once

* Leslie Walker-Hirsch and Marklyn P. Champagne, "The Circles Concept: Social Competence in Special Education," *Contemporary Issues—Sexuality Education* (Sept. 1991): 65–67.

the circles are established, it's time for the big question: how do you keep the information inside its own circle and prevent it from leaking to people in an outer ring? The answer is, of course, that you *can't* absolutely keep that from happening. You can certainly create stopgaps and systems to minimize leakage, but once you release information into any of the circles besides the innermost one that contains only you, you've lost control of it. That's why it's so important to carefully consider who is in each circle and what information you want to share with them.

I like this exercise because it helps kids understand that they have control over what people do and do not know about them, but *only if* they define and enforce their own privacy policies. One of the ways in which we keep our information private is to maintain clear boundaries between the concentric circles. How do you keep things in that inner circle and what are the consequences if private information leaks out? It's important for your kids to see that what seems like a simple text can have ripple effects on their lives. Would your child want to face classmates after everyone saw a nude photo of them? If a racy text is sent out to a kid's broader circle of friends, will it change those friendships? What if their teachers or friends' parents see it? How might it change those relationships, and how might it influence the way your child feels about themself?

For example, if a person takes a naked or partially naked selfie and sends it to three people in their innermost circle, how likely is it that the photo will stay in that inner circle? Even if a teen's closest friend shows it to only one other person, then all of those barriers between the circles can break down. The illusion of control is lost. If your secret can get out of the inner circle, then it can get out of any circle. As soon as the walls are penetrated, the circles disintegrate, and there's no reason why a complete stranger couldn't see the picture of your body. And that can lead to harassment, bullying, and college officials and employers seeing things online that will damage a kid's future.

What ups the ante in the lives of today's teens is the speed at which kids can share online material. Even a decade ago, if you gave a sexy photograph of yourself to your sweetheart, it might have been passed around the school, sure. But there would have been time to contain it, to find out who had it and demand the photo's return. You could have ripped it up into pieces and buried it in your backyard. Kids today aren't so lucky. Now a provocative photo sent electronically can be passed to dozens of kids within seconds. It gets to those outermost privacy circles faster than a child can run a lap on the track. Some kids think using Snapchat, an app that allows you to upload a photo, share it, and have it vanish after ten seconds, is a way to maintain privacy. In the same breath, though, they'll admit there's a way around the ten-second delete—take a screen shot of the pic so you have it forever.

My students report that sexting among their peers mostly happens between romantic partners. It would be wrong to assume that every teenager in a relationship sexts, though—I think there are plenty of kids who don't feel comfortable being that explicit with their sweethearts. For those who do sext, I have to think that part of it comes from wanting to feel closer to their partners—and because part of loving people is trusting them, sometimes this kind of electronic bonding can give students a false sense of security about maintaining private information. They trust that their sweethearts aren't going to show the pictures or sexually charged texts to anyone, but what if they do? I also challenge my students to think about what happens to the texts or photos after a breakup. We would hope that an ex would maintain a former sweetheart's privacy. But what if there's a person inside a sweetheart's inner circle who isn't in one's *own* inner circle?

There's also something called *revenge porn*. This is when after a fight or a breakup, someone shares a photo or text that was sent privately as a way of "getting back" at the partner who made them angry or broke up with them. Revenge porn is an especially egregious form of betrayal because it deliberately violates expectations of privacy that were previously established. The legal system has taken notice of increasing incidents of revenge porn and laws are being passed to make the behavior illegal, but those laws aren't universal and they don't guarantee the behavior will stop.

Whether your child is in a relationship or not, you can easily start the conversation with a "why" and a "what if." Why would you take a provocative picture of your body in the first place? What's the motivation behind it? Did your sweetheart ask you to do it? Is it because "everybody's" doing it? Are you just curious to see what it will look like? Once you take a provocative photo or video of your body, how would you ensure that it's going to stay with the people you sent it to? What are your options, if it's sent to someone else?

In the early days of the HIV/AIDS pandemic, we used to tell people to assume that everyone they were engaging in high-risk behaviors with *was* HIV-positive, because the best way to protect yourself was to take universal precautions instead of judging each experience on a case-by-case basis. That same lesson applies to digital privacy—a blanket rule should apply. I tell kids to assume that anything they put online can and will be seen by everyone else who is able to go online. Universal precautions are still the best way to maintain safety.

I know that my words will not stop every kid from sexting, so I also offer what I call some tips for "safer sexting." I make it clear that I don't want them to sext at all; that I think it's a dangerous and foolish behavior. But, if they are determined to do it, I also want to help them minimize the potential damage that can be done. One can minimize damage by being able to say convincingly, "That's not me." So, how can a person create plausible deniability when sexting? I start with the students saying they won't put their face in the photo or video, and I think that's very smart, but they also need to think about any unique body markings they have (tattoos, birthmarks, scars, etc.). Those need to remain out of view too. Further, what's the background of the photo or video? If everyone knows what your bedroom or your living room looks like, that's another way to connect the photo to you. What account or phone number is the photo being sent from? If it's clearly from your e-mail address or cell phone number, it's linked to you. Students see quickly that it can be quite difficult to distance themselves from a sext.

A bigger problem is that many young people don't want to hide their identity. A recent phenomena is OnlyFans, an online service where individuals can post nude or sexually explicit videos of themselves that others can subscribe to and view. In theory only a subscriber who pays money to the content creator can see what's posted, but that's hardly a guarantee of privacy. Consenting adults may freely choose something like OnlyFans as a means of generating income, but minors using this platform is problematic if not illegal.

....

I wish there were "dumb" phones for parents to buy their younger kids. They would look like smartphones, but they'd allow you to make calls and send texts only to preset numbers. Kids wouldn't have wide-open access to the Internet, and they wouldn't be able to send or receive e-mails, share photos, or access social media from their phones. Parents can and should set boundaries about smartphone and computer use, but the truth is kids can type anything into a search engine and get hundreds of results at their fingertips. Statistics show that kids are getting phones around age ten or eleven, and according to data from Statista.com, in 2019, 65 percent of children got their first cell phone between ages nine and fourteen (19.2 percent between nine and ten; 25.7 percent between eleven and twelve; 20.5 percent between thirteen and fourteen). The same data showed that a full 16 percent of children were getting access to their first cell phone before the age of seven!* It's difficult for parents to talk to teens about sex, let alone younger children. But it's becoming clear that conversations about sexting and establishing and maintaining online privacy need to start taking place earlier and earlier.

Most middle-school children are fully online. At this age, I

....

* S. O'Dea, "What Age Are Kids When Parents First Buy/Give Them Their Own Cell Phone?" Statista, October 19, 2021, https://www.statista.com/statistics/1058938/cell-phone-owhnership-among-children-in-the-us-by-age/.

think it's extremely important to keep tabs on what your child is doing online and to establish clear boundaries and full transparency when it comes to social media, e-mail, and even texting. Parents should have *full* access to these accounts at all times. That means that you should be able to see your child's friend list, status updates, and private messages. That doesn't mean you'll constantly be snooping, but it does mean your child knows that part of the deal with their digital access is that *you* have access to all of their online information, and that can be an important factor in helping them make good decisions. It's perfectly reasonable to scroll through your child's text messages or e-mails at the end of the day or on a weekly basis—and do it *with* your child. Show your kids that you're interested in only their safety and you're not trying to ruin their lives. Don't feel sheepish or skittish. You are responsible for their safety—they're still children, and as much as they think they know everything, they are incredibly vulnerable. It's our job to use a heavy hand in helping them navigate this new world they're encountering. If you see something you think is inappropriate, don't yell or take the phone away. Use the opportunity as a way into some of these conversations about privacy. Make every moment a teachable moment.

When kids leave middle school and grow into the high school years, parents find themselves in a delicate dance when it comes to accessing their kids' social media accounts and cell phones. As liberal a sex educator as I am, I still think it's reasonable for parents to have access to their teen's devices and social media accounts, especially if they're the ones paying for them. Once a teen is able to pay for their own devices and connection charges, then it's theirs to manage on their own. If an adult is looking through a teen's device, here's what's not OK—reacting with punishment to anything you find. For instance, let's say you scroll through text messages and see that your child has been cursing up a storm or saying inappropriate things about (or to) their sweetheart. This is not the time to yell and punish your kid for bad language. If a clear boundary had been set—don't send texts with curse words—and it has been violated, that's different. But if you suddenly yell at your children for things said in a private conversation, they're going to resent you and most likely trust you less. Kids break rules; they push boundaries—and language is one way they experiment with that. It's part of being a kid. When parents jump to conclusions or anger rather than teachable moments, they open a chasm between them and their kid, which is the last thing you want with an already aloof (or private or mysterious) teenager.

Ideally, we want teens to be able to self-regulate and make healthy decisions about privacy. Kids don't learn how to do that unless we give them a chance to try. Mistakes will be made. That's part of growing up. Our job is to try to minimize those mistakes (and the long-term impact of them) for our kids. That's the great thing about high school. You can screw up, but it doesn't ruin the rest of your life. Your kids won't be perfect. But instead of feeling helpless and fearing the worst, stay informed, stay calm, and keep the lines of communication open.

....

Neither cell phones nor computers nor pocket calculators are evil; they're tools. They don't cause the ruination of children any more than a hammer does. Sure, if you don't know how to use a hammer, you can end up hurting yourself or someone else. In skilled hands, though, a hammer can be used to create everything from a solid structure in which to live to a beautiful piece of art. What makes the difference is knowledge, training, and, yes, experience. The same is true for any technological device. By forbidding my brother and me from using his pocket calculator, my father made it more likely that if we did come upon one, as was inevitable, we'd be ill equipped to use it well. Like everything else we've talked about in this book, the keys to success for your children's use of technology are clear communication, setting and reinforcing limits when appropriate, and most important, aiming for the good outcome rather than planning for the disastrous one.

....

Question Box

Q: Why are guys so obsessed with boobs?

A: The simple answer is because they've been taught to be obsessed with breasts. Not every culture sees women's breasts as a focus for sexual pleasure or attraction. What tends to make breasts the object of sexual desire is not seeing them regularly in a society. In societies where women routinely go topless, breasts are seen as just another body part. Some will find them sexually stimulating, others will not. In the United States, however, women's breasts are not routinely visible. That can make them become an object of desire. It's clear that in this country we make a strong connection between women's breasts and sex. Once a culture makes this connection, then women's breasts become more and more sexualized and take on greater importance. Guys are told they *must* be interested in women's breasts—that such an interest is part of being a man. This is unfair both to men and to women. It creates all this drama around a body part that in other situations might just be allowed to be one part among many others—as men's breasts are in this country. Also note that women and nonbinary people can also be turned on by women's breasts. It's not only about what men feel.

Q: Is the term *blue balls* (when you don't ejaculate for a period of time and your balls turn blue) a real thing?

A: The answer to this question is both yes and no, so let's explore it in detail.

When a person is sexually excited, blood rushes into their entire genital area. For guys that includes the penis, scrotum, and testes. For girls it includes the vulva and area around the vagina. As long as sexual excitement continues, the blood will get held there. If a person stays in a state of sexual excitement for a long time, it's just like trying to hold a yoga pose or hold up a set of weights for a long time: Your body gets fatigued from that exertion. So it's possible that a guy's testes can start to feel sore and achy during prolonged sexual excitement. But, they don't turn blue—and even if they did (which they don't) how would you see that? Testes are inside the scrotum, remember? Last time I checked, scrotums don't have see-through windows or little doors that you can open to look inside them.

Now here's the REALLY important thing about blue balls. For decades guys have told their sexual partners that it's dangerous (maybe even deadly) to have blue balls, and the only solution is for the partner to help the guy have an orgasm and/or ejaculation. THAT'S A LIE! Blue balls may be uncomfortable but it's not dangerous or deadly and there are PLENTY of ways to get relief. Yes, an orgasm and ejaculation will do it, but that's not the only way! If you were holding a yoga pose or a set of weights too long and you got achy, what would you do? You'd release the pose or the weights and relax. That's all a person has to do when they're achy from prolonged sexual excitement. Give yourself a minute to relax, let the blood flow out of that genital area for a minute or two, and then you're good to go again.

Q: Is lube necessary during sex or is it just helpful?

A: This question seems pretty simple, but depending on what kind of sex we're talking about, the answer changes.

If the sex is vaginal intercourse, the answer is "It depends." The vagina is self-lubricating. During sexual excitement, it secretes a fluid that serves as a natural lubricant. You may have heard about a female bodied person "getting wet"—that's what they're talking about. This vaginal lubrication is the first sign of sexual excitement in a female bodied person (just like an erection is the first sign of sexual excitement in a male bodied person). While all vaginas lubricate when excited, the amount of lubrication varies. Sometimes it's more than enough to make intercourse pleasurable and sometimes it's not. It's always a good idea to have a water-based lubricant on hand for vaginal intercourse. There are a lot of things that can interfere with the amount of natural lubrication a person produces, including if a person is nervous. Vaginal intercourse shouldn't hurt. If it is hurting the person being penetrated, then more lubrication may be the answer.

If the sex is anal intercourse, always use lots of lube. The anus does not have any self-lubricating mechanism, so adding lubricant protects the thin, delicate anal lining from tearing during intercourse. Anal intercourse shouldn't hurt. If it is hurting the person being penetrated, more lubrication is needed.

You will see that there are different kinds of lubricants: water-based, oil-based, or silicone-based. Water-based lubricants are the most common and can be used whether or not the penetrating partner is using a condom (although condoms should always be used for intercourse activities). Water-based lube needs to be reapplied often, so keep it handy and don't be afraid to use more of it if it starts to dry. Oil-based lubricants will damage latex condoms so they should be avoided. Silicone-based lubricants are harder to find, but they are good to use because they are more slippery than water-based lubricants and don't need to be reapplied as often.

Short answer: Lube is always helpful and often necessary!

Q: So I'm in a secret relationship (I'm an underclassman and he's an upperclassman) and he really wants to go public with our relationship, but I just don't think it's a good idea. He's looking at colleges and I really don't want to hold him back. What should I do?

A: First, secret relationships are ALWAYS trouble. What's the reason for keeping the relationship secret? Who is being protected? What harm would come if the relationship was public? I can't see any reason for a relationship, especially one between a younger person and an older person, to remain a secret.

Second, relationships between ninth-graders and eleventh- or twelfth-graders are usually trouble. There's a huge imbalance of power in a relationship between a ninth- or tenth-grader and an eleventh- or twelfth-grader, and that imbalance of power can lead to the younger person being taken advantage of in big and small ways.

To answer your specific question, in my mind the relationship HAS to go public. Keeping it a secret is not an option. You have zero chance of holding him back from college—he's going to go and your relationship will end or change when that happens. That's just the way high school relationships work. And going public means it has to be all the way public. Your parents, his parents, your friends, and his friends all have to know about the relationship. If you feel like you can't tell your family or friends about the relationship, that raises serious questions about whether being in the relationship is a good idea in the first place.

....

CHAPTER 9

"Lights! Camera! Conversation!": Let's Talk About Pornography.

A student came up to me after class, looking to make sure his classmates weren't in earshot.

"Mr. V," he asked quietly, "it's not bad to look at porn, is it?"

"I know the answer you want by the way you asked the question," I said.

"Well, yeah," he said, "I mean, it's not *bad*, right?"

"It doesn't *have* to be, but it *can* be. Can I ask you a couple of questions?"

"Sure," he mumbled, looking more sorry by the minute that he brought this up.

"What's the way we defined 'having sex' in the lesson we had last week?" I asked.

"Conditions are more important than behaviors, right?" he half said, half asked.

"Right!" I said. "And what conditions did we say were important to having healthy sex?"

It took him a minute, but he remembered them: "Consensual,

sober, mutually pleasurable, has the chance for connection or intimacy, and people aren't treated as objects."

"Awesome job!" I said a bit too loudly. A couple of kids looked our way. I had to bring my volume down to continue. "So, how sure are you porn fits those conditions?"

"I'm consenting to watch it. I get pleasure from it. I was sober when I watched it." I noticed he stopped there and ignored the rest of the list.

"Yeah, I'm not really asking about you, though." I prodded. "What about the people performing in the porn? Can you be sure the conditions were met for them?"

"I don't know," he said glumly.

"I don't know either," I said. "So you see, the answer to your question is more complex than a simple yes or no."

"It always is with you," he said. He didn't walk away satisfied, but he wasn't mad either. He was thinking. I consider that a win.

....

Talking about healthy sexuality with young people absolutely entails talking to them about Internet pornography. Accessing pornography today is much different than it was "back in the day." My students simultaneously howl with laughter and cringe when I tell them that in precomputer days getting porn required a face-to-face interaction. You actually had to walk up to the counter in the video store and say to the person standing there that, yes, this is the video you wanted to rent. It was anything but an anonymous transaction. A young man I know well (and I'll say no more than that) thought that he was slick, and always rented a film he considered "highbrow" along with the porn video—you know, so the person at the register wouldn't think he was just some pervert. He rented *A Fish Called Wanda* about twenty times (which also suggests he wasn't very adept at knowing what a highbrow film was), and to this day I . . . he . . . can't tell you a thing about that movie.

Today many young people will access pornography, often unintentionally, simply because it's so easily available on the Web—so it's important that what they see is given some context. According to Culture Reframed, an organization dedicated to pointing out the problems with the mainstream pornography industry, porn sites get more visitors each month than Netflix, Amazon, and Twitter combined. PornHub alone, which describes itself as "the world's leading free porn site," had forty-two billion visits in 2019. Now we can't say what percentage of the visitors to these sites are young people, but what number, if any, would make you feel OK?

For many teens and preteens, porn offers their first view of what sexual activity looks like. Unfortunately, it offers some very unhealthy messages. One is that sex is the entirety of life. Every interaction is just a prelude to sexual activity, and every interaction leads to and is centered on sex. Healthy sexuality means being able to integrate the fact that we are beings who desire and have sexual activity into lives that are often decidedly unsexy. How many of you have been faced with a burst pipe in your house? When the plumber arrives, no matter how sexy they may be, you want the pipe fixed, but not in porn! There's a time and place for sexual activity in a whole, healthy, fulfilling life. When we compartmentalize our sexual lives we often develop shame and guilt around them. That's not seeing our sexuality and our sexual capacities as a force for good in the world.

Another set of unhealthy messages from porn deal with how they portray women. A lot of mainstream, heterosexual pornography is very degrading toward women. Women are used purely as sex objects by the men in the film. This can make someone think those kinds of attitudes and behaviors toward women are OK, and they never are. Some pornography incorporates a lot of violence, especially against women. It has been shown that those who watch violent pornography have more lenient attitudes about things like sexual harassment and even rape in the real world. Watching something over and over normalizes it in our brains and we can become numb to its effects.

Finally, mainstream pornography is largely based on heterosexual interactions among white able-bodied people. When it does portray different ethnicities, orientations, abilities, etc., it often does so in a fetishizing way. This goes against one of my goals as a sexuality educator—to foster and promote healthy human sexuality that recognizes the many ways race, class, ethnicity, orientation, ability, and other human diversity enhance human dignity. Pornography has a poor record of meeting this goal.

I've done some work with Culture Reframed, and what I appreciate about the organization is that they understand the real problem with mainstream porn. It's listed right on their website: "In the absence of comprehensive, competent sex education, porn serves as the major form of sex ed for millions of kids. And what are kids learning? That degradation, humiliation, and violence are central to relationships, intimacy, and sex." What about those kids who *do* get age-appropriate, progressive, comprehensive sexuality education, or who have adults in their lives who are willing to talk with them calmly and nonjudgmentally? They are much more equipped to see porn for what it is and push back against the negative messages it offers. So when we ignore porn, we allow it to become the teacher for our teens (and children). Our kids deserve better, so we have to step up and speak up. Let's talk about how we can do that.

When I talk about pornography in my classes, I don't start with accusations like, "I know you're all watching porn!" That's not true, and it immediately puts kids on the defensive. Instead, I start with naming the reality of our society today. "We're going to talk about pornography. I'm not assuming you're looking at it or not. That's none of my business, and I'm not going to ask you about that. But porn is a fact of life in our world today. It's easy to find, and we need to be smart about it. Pretending it doesn't exist or that we're not the kind of people who would watch that stuff is naive. So, let's be real, OK?"

Can you imagine starting a conversation with your kid with words like that? Why not practice coming up with your own introduction? Just remember: don't accuse, inform. What if you know your child has been looking at online porn? You can be honest about that without being accusatory. "I want to talk with you about some of the things you've been looking at online. I'm not going to yell, and I'm not going to put you down. I just want to share a few things I know about pornography because I want to make sure you know them too."

Pornography versus Sexually Explicit Material

The first point I make when talking about pornography is to draw a distinction between pornography and what I call "sexually explicit material." One of the traps we can fall into as well-meaning adults who want to protect kids is to classify anything that has to do with nudity, sexual activity, or sexuality in general as porn. That's neither true nor helpful in this conversation. Pornography is material designed to sexually stimulate or excite. It's made for prurient interests. *Prurient* is a great word. Merriam-Webster defines it as, "marked by or arousing an immoderate or unwholesome interest or desire." It's material that exists mainly to turn people on, to be salacious, maybe even crude. I define sexually explicit material as: material designed to educate or inform, not to excite. Think about that distinction; it's an important one. Anatomical drawings of genitals are sexually explicit, but are they pornographic? Is explaining how an erection happens by using a drawing or even a photo of an erect penis pornographic? I'd say no. A series of pictures that shows how to insert and remove a tampon or how to put a condom on a penis is sexually explicit, but it's not designed to turn anyone on. A picture of a mother breastfeeding her baby isn't porn. I have a great drawing that is so heavily anatomically labeled that kids struggle to figure out what it is. After looking at it for a while, they realize it's showing a cross section of a male and female body with an erect penis inside a vagina. I then reveal the heading at the top of the drawing. It says "Sexual Intercourse." So there I am, showing my kids an actual drawing of the act of sexual intercourse.

"Pretty sexy, huh?" I say to the class, giving them a slightly sly look. None of them think so.

Now I'm not saying a person *can't* be turned on by any of this material. Humans have an amazing capacity to be sexually excited by all kinds of things, but none of these materials are made with the intention of stimulating or exciting the viewer. Pornography is. So, think about what you would do in this situation: A young person is curious about bodies and sex. They don't have easy access to any material that shows them that except for pornography. They access porn to learn the different ways naked human bodies can look, and to figure out what this thing called "sex" is. They're not seeking out something to masturbate with; they're just curious in a way that's perfectly natural and age appropriate.

How do we approach this kid? How do we start that conversation? How and when *does* one learn that there's such a thing as a penis going inside a vagina? How does one understand what that means? Without conversation and context it's all gibberish. One of the things we have to make clear to kids is that their curiosity isn't wrong. We also have to give them resources that can help them satisfy their curiosity in ways that won't harm them.

For younger children, the website Amaze.org has wonderful, short, cartoon videos that give age-appropriate information about bodies, sexuality, sexual activity, consent, diversity, you name it! It's a website I'd feel very comfortable letting a middle school or high school student peruse at will. The website has videos that are appropriate for even younger kids. I select some of the videos to use with our fourth- and fifth-graders during our classes on puberty and crushes. For teenagers, websites like Sex, Etc.; Scarleteen; and Guerilla Sex Ed are excellent resources to find out all kinds of information about healthy bodies and healthy sexuality—and they're all perfectly appropriate for adolescents. Much of the content on Sex, Etc. and Scarleteen are written by teens themselves.

Pornography isn't the only option, and it's nowhere close to the best option, to satisfy a young person's natural curiosity about sex. But if we don't tell them that, how will they know?

What Can Pornography Do?

An activity I do in class with my students is based upon an excellent lesson plan from the curriculum *Streetwise and Sexwise* by Steve Brown. This manual and many other fantastic sexuality education curricula are published by the Center for Sex Education. The activity gives students a series of statements and asks them if they think pornography accomplishes that. Kids can answer "yes," "no," or "maybe." Anyone can respond to these statements, whether they have viewed pornographic materials or not, and, as with all activities, participation is voluntary and students can choose whether or not to respond to each statement. Here are the statements I use:

1. Pornography shows possible ways of achieving pleasure.
2. Pornography shows how to talk in advance about sex with a partner.
3. Pornography shows various types of sexual behavior.
4. Pornography shows how to start a sexual relationship with someone.
5. Pornography shows how to say no to unwanted sexual behavior.
6. Pornography shows how to have an orgasm.
7. Pornography shows what average people's bodies and sexual organs look like.
8. Pornography shows safer sex practices for preventing pregnancy and STIs.

9. Pornography shows sex involving an emotional connection with another person.
10. Pornography shows how long sexual activity typically takes.

The noise level in the classroom rises as students discuss and debate the statements. Some argue that pornography *could* do any of these things. Before I can step in, they're challenged by their classmates to think about what pornography *usually* does or is *intended* to do. Many students have never thought about the purposes or intentions of pornography. It simply exists as a reality in their world. At the end of the activity some clear "no"s emerge. The class pretty much agrees that pornography doesn't show how to talk in advance about sex, or start a sexual relationship, or say no to unwanted sex, or show how to use safer sex practices. A lot of their answers to the other statements are "maybe." Pornography seems to show people having orgasms and engaging in various kinds of sexual behavior, and sometimes it seems like the people in the scene have an emotional connection. This is where it's essential to remind kids of one of the most important facts about pornography. It's acting; it's a performance.

The people in a pornographic movie are well aware that they're not performing for each other but for their audience. It's not actually a secret window into the real world. It's a completely constructed world, as fake as any movie on the big screen or any "reality" show they stream on their laptops. Our kids grow up in a media-saturated world and can actually be quite savvy consumers, but they don't make the connection that pornography is just another medium that is highly scripted and produced.

When your kids watch a box-office blockbuster that appears to be one seamless progression of events, they know that it's actually the result of many different cuts strung together. A movie is not filmed start to finish. The scenes are filmed out of order and cut together to make what looks like a coherent whole. The same is true in porn. The orgasm may be filmed before the kissing. What looks like uninterrupted sex may be filmed over a number of days. Even if it is all filmed at one time, those people aren't having uninterrupted sex for hours. They're starting and stopping, resetting cameras, having their makeup fixed, dealing with technical glitches, and the like.

When we watch our favorite action hero jump through an explosion and come out unscathed, we're aware on some level that it's an illusion, and this is what we need kids to realize about pornography. Also, because it's filmed for an audience and not for the private enjoyment of the performers, the sexual activities the people engage in might not be the ones they would choose. They're chosen for them based on what someone thinks the audience wants to see. The pleasure that appears to be real might just be skillful acting; anyone can be taught to moan and look like something is fun, even when it may not be. And, yes, orgasms, no matter who is having them, can be faked.

This line of discussion allows me to bring up some other points that I want students to think about. Pornography is a business, and it's fair to state that as a fact. So, I ask students, "Why do you think someone decides to go into the porn industry (not as an actor, but into the business of making and distributing porn)? What's their primary goal? What rules do the businesspeople in porn have to follow? Who regulates them?"

My students are clear that people go into producing porn to make money. The other questions are trickier for them. They don't know anything about how the industry might be regulated or whether it's completely unregulated. That's not typically what they're searching for when they're looking up pornography on the Internet.

It's important teens know that mainstream pornography is a business that makes billions of dollars every year. Like many other businesses, owners focus on profits often at the expense of people (actors or viewers). I then make a connection that can make them uncomfortable. This is not unlike a lot of the big companies that make sneakers or clothes. How often do we think about the conditions under which workers make those things? How often do we think about how buying them impacts us or them? How often do we know that our sneakers or jeans are made in sweatshops around the world that exploit its laborers, but don't care?

When it comes to thinking about the actors in mainstream porn, I want students to consider whether they've entered into the pornography industry willingly and eagerly. Are they paid fairly for their work? Do they get health benefits? Do they get screened for STIs? Do they have a retirement plan? Do the actors have good working conditions?

Many students assume that everyone in porn wants to be there and is OK with what they're doing. They may not be familiar with the idea of survival sex—exchanging sex to meet one's immediate needs, like food, shelter, child care, etc. Sometimes this is done out of desperation, sometimes it's done in addition to other low-paying work that does not allow a person to earn a living wage. Students often assume that actors in the porn industry get a lot of money for the work they do. That's not true. There are a small handful of performers, mostly women, who make large sums of money; most make small amounts—maybe a few hundred dollars for a scene. The mainstream pornography industry has a poor track record of taking care of the people who perform in it. There is a lot of exploitation of young people, women, men, and nonbinary folks in the industry. Not everyone who is appearing in pornography has entered into it eagerly and willingly. Not everyone is being paid fairly. It's hard to know whether that's true or not for any individual instance of pornography that a person watches.

There is an excellent film available on Netflix called *Hot Girls Wanted*. It isn't pornographic; it's a documentary that made huge waves at the 2015 Sundance Film Festival. It follows young women who answer ads that promise them freedom, money, and opportunity in the porn industry. It's an eye-opening look at the industry from the inside. What it shows is not pretty or glamorous, but neither is it sensational. It's real, and it's just the dose of reality our young people may need to begin to understand and humanize the young people who often enter the porn industry based on promises that are never delivered.

I also always ask this question when we're talking about the actors in pornography. "What do you imagine the people in those porn scenes are doing twenty minutes after the camera stops? Are they grocery shopping? Are they checking their cell phones? Are they still having sex?" My students usually don't have an answer to the question; no one's ever asked them that before. It's easy to believe that porn stars exist in a sex bubble, that they always live in that warehouse or bedroom or on that pool deck. They don't think about the fact that there's more to life than sex because porn depicts only the sexual selves. It's really easy to forget about all of the complexities of being human in the lives of the people you're watching. It can be harder for people to watch porn when they think about the actors as real people who have parents, families, laundry, or homework to do—so pornography erases all that unless it's in the service of the sex they want to portray.

"You're ruining porn, Mr. V!" a young man groans. He's wearing a team jersey and is a highly valued athlete at school. He's also a sensitive kid who has a big heart and I know I've struck a nerve with him. His protest is almost a plea not to make him have to think about or feel these things.

"That's not my intention, really!" I protest. "But I do want you to think about the reality of the industry and the people in it."

"But that ruins it!", the young man snaps back. "It's supposed to be a fantasy, and you say fantasy is OK!"

"I absolutely do say that, and I stand by it," I say as I smile and point to him. "Look at what you just said, it's *supposed* to be a fantasy. Some things can live purely in the realm of fantasy, like fan fiction or cartoons or novels or even erotic stories, but in porn people are the products being sold. We can't forget that."

"I can try," the young man says, his eyes downcast.

What About "Amateur Porn"?

The pornography our kids consume today isn't all highly produced, scripted, "professional" porn. I talked about OnlyFans in the last chapter, but you don't have to go to pay sites like that to find amateur porn. Did you know that Twitter, Tumblr, and to some degree even TikTok are loaded with porn along their other

content? Anyone with a cell phone or a computer can send themselves out to the world where there is a willing audience ready
to watch. Many teens have taken nude photos of themselves or
their genitals, and many have filmed themselves masturbating or
engaging in sexual activity with someone else. Talk to kids today
and you may find to your horror that this isn't fringe behavior;
it's pretty mainstream. We all crave attention, no more so than
when we're adolescents desperate for approval and confirmation
that we're OK.

"Would you want someone to watch you have sex?" I ask my
students one day.

"You mean, like, in real life or on video?" a student asks.

"Either," I say.

"Eww, creepy," says a girl in sweats and a ponytail. A boy next
to her shrugs.

"Talk to me about the difference between someone actually
being there watching you have sex and someone watching you do
it on a video," I nudge.

"The person standing there watching is obviously a perv!" says
a guy in a college sweatshirt and baseball cap. "But watching it on
video is just . . . I dunno . . . different. I think that's OK."

"But it's still you," I push back, "whether in person or on screen.
Someone you don't know is watching you in a pretty vulnerable
moment." I'm not going to win this one, and I know it. Many of
my students don't see the connection between what happens in
real time and what happens on the screen. It's troubling to me,
and I have to remind myself yet again that I didn't grow up in this
always-online world, and my ideas of privacy are very different
from theirs. As a last resort I try to make the point that we live

and act in the real world, not the virtual world. Just because you can watch real people having sex on a screen does not mean you are ready, skilled, or knowledgeable about what having sex in the real world is like. They're not meant to be "how-to" videos.

I try to show that the same performative aspect we talk about in mainstream porn exists in "amateur" porn. When you film yourself naked or masturbating or having sex, you do it because you want someone else to see it. You have to ask, "How does the presence of a camera change a sexual interaction, whether solo or between two or more people?" Isn't it likely that people are going to do things and say things they don't normally do or say, even things that might not be true, because it's part of their performance? If you totally forget the camera is there, you get a lousy product that no one wants to watch.

Amateur pornography involving minors is especially troubling. I always remind my students that our legal system tends to lag behind what's become more normalized in our society. Laws about child pornography are very strict and unforgiving, and they should be. Taking a photo of a nude minor or a minor in a sexual encounter is seen by the law as creating child pornography. Sharing such a photo or video is distributing child pornography. These activities can have incredibly heavy consequences, and the law doesn't always make allowances for youthful indiscretions or mistakes—and ignorance of the law is no excuse for violating it.

Think about what this means. We have a huge number of kids who, while still minors themselves, are making and distributing something that can legally qualify as child pornography. We have to make sure they know that. As we talked about in the last chapter, sexting is a common practice among romantic partners, and revenge porn is an ever-growing practice. It's unlikely that sexting between teenagers is going to wind up in a court of law, but no one can guarantee that. Many of the seniors in my Sexuality and Society class are eighteen or will turn eighteen during the school year. The law changes after that, but some of them have sweethearts that aren't yet eighteen.

Please be careful how you talk about this with teens who are still legally minors. Don't tell them that if they sext or make amateur porn that they're going to go to jail. That's fearmongering, not education. Fear-based tactics are lousy at creating lasting behavior change, and they don't lead to the kind of open and trusting communication we're trying to establish. This is one important point among many that we want kids to think about when it comes to pornography. It's a difficult point because it is scary, and it also flies in the face of what many teens see every day. Still, we need to talk about it calmly and place it alongside the other messages we want to convey. Don't lead with it, but don't bury it either.

OK, So Can I Watch It or Not?

By the end of our discussions about pornography, many of my students' heads are spinning. They've been confronted with a lot of new information and they need time to process it. It's pretty common that a deeply frustrated voice finally asks the question:

"So, just tell us. Can we watch porn or not?!"

As usual, I have somewhat of an answer and a whole lot more questions:

"The answer isn't the same for every person, and it depends on some essential questions: What's the main reason a person your age views pornography? How does a viewer know if porn is having a negative or damaging effect on them?"

I tell students that, when it comes to viewing pornography, how one responds to and is affected by it can vary greatly. It's important for the viewer to think about what impact viewing pornography is having on their lives, both their sexual lives and their nonsexual lives. One might think about who they choose to tell about their pornography viewing. Is it a completely hidden part of one's life? Is it something one can talk about with friends or family? Is it something one wants to be known for? Why or why not? The decision whether to view pornography or not is a personal one. Like all decisions we talk about in my class, it should be made thoughtfully and deliberately. It should be a decision that is in line with one's values and that one can defend if challenged.

One final point I want to talk about is the idea of becoming addicted to pornography. I purposely don't use the word *addiction* when talking to students about porn use. I do this for two reasons. First, I haven't seen enough evidence in peer-reviewed scientific journals that show pornography's effect on the brain is similar to alcohol or other illicit substances. There's plenty of information online that claims it does the same thing as alcohol, but the sources of that information don't hold up for me. The second reason I avoid the word *addiction* is that it's too scary a word to use with my high school students. They know what addiction is. Many of them have seen people in their lives live with, struggle with, and work to overcome addiction. Some of my students have done this themselves. The concept of addiction sets up a seemingly insurmountable task for many kids. It shuts down conversation where I'm trying to open it up.

Instead of *addiction*, I use the word *habit*. Watching pornography can become a habit, and habits can certainly get out of control. Habits, however, unlike addiction, can be broken and changed without needing extraordinary means. One of the problems with habits is that once we habituate doing something, we don't really think about what we're doing; the behavior just becomes automatic. This can pose several problems. Some people find that because they only masturbate while watching pornography, it becomes difficult to masturbate or achieve an orgasm in other ways, including when with a partner. Here a person is not only habitualizing watching porn, they're habitualizing their masturbation habit as well. I've seen many a spark of recognition in the eyes of students when talking about this.

Some people's pornography habit gets in the way of other important things in their life. People who can't get their schoolwork done because they just keep watching porn instead or who are isolating from friends or family have a problematic porn habit that needs attention. Some people find that watching pornography gets boring. They seek out more intense or unusual forms of porn to try to get restimulated. Since very few people in the real world engage in these extreme behaviors, this can cause problems when these people are seeking out real sexual partners. Talking about porn as a habit encourages young people to think about how they might alter their own behavior to bring their life more into alignment with the people they want to be. Of course there is a place for adults to help in this process, especially when a young person is having difficulty changing a habit that's particularly stubborn. I'm not saying they have to do it alone, but I want to empower them to take ownership of their own behaviors because that's an important step in becoming a healthy adult.

....

If we think of pornography as just another kind of media, I maintain that if you can talk with your kids about a TV show, music video, movie, or YouTube video, you can talk to them about porn. You don't even have to have seen the specific porn your kids might be viewing, or any porn, for that matter. Remember, often kids look to porn to help them figure out what sex is like, but they get a totally skewed picture. Our role, as always, is to provide context. Porn is not like real-life sex, and the earlier that kids learn that, the healthier the relationships they'll be able to carry on. While trying hard to convey the message that porn isn't real, we also have to be clear that the messages porn sends about women, about sex, about violence—and especially about the interaction of all those—are very real and can be very damaging. Our kids aren't just internalizing messages about what sex is like when they watch porn uncritically; they're also internalizing very skewed messages about what it means to be a man or a woman, about the place of violence in sexual activity, and about how dehumanizing sex can be. None of those messages are healthy ones, so we have to be able to counter them.

Question Box

Q: Do you think pornography encourages the baseball model?

A: I absolutely think pornography encourages the baseball model. It highlights vaginal intercourse over other kinds of sexual activity, and it often promotes the idea of the "bases" as the actors go through a series of regulated steps in their sexual activity—moving from kissing to touching to oral sex to vaginal intercourse. You can't get more "baseball" than that!

Pornography is also problematic because it gives unrealistic models of what sexual activity is really like, reinforces very rigid and traditional gender roles, and promotes unrealistic body images (especially for women).

Honestly, I don't think pornography can be considered a part of healthy sexuality for high school-age students. Pornography is another form of media, just like TV, and TV gives us mostly unhealthy models of sexuality and sexual activity. Viewing pornography on a regular basis can fill a person's head with many unrealistic expectations of what sexual activity may be like. Those unrealistic expectations can mess people up when they encounter real-life sexual situations. If a young person is going to view pornography (and, as I said above, I don't think that's necessarily healthy), please be clear that this material represents *unrealistic fantasies*. There is nothing about the way pornography portrays sexual activity that translates in "real" life. The clearer you are about that, the better off you'll be.

Here's another thing you probably never thought about. What

do you think those actors and actresses do after they're finished filming a scene? Pornography causes us to dehumanize the people involved in it. We don't think of them as real people, but they are. We're real people too, so our lives can't be about sex twenty-four hours a day, seven days a week either. When would you get your homework done?

Q: Is it normal that I'm not into pornography but I do masturbate? I am male.

A: It's absolutely normal! The idea that every guy will be into viewing pornography is a stereotype. The same goes for the stereotype that all girls aren't into viewing porn. Some guys and girls like to watch it, others don't. Some people use pornography while masturbating, others don't. The important thing is that you do whatever feels most natural and right for you.

Q: Why is watching pornography such a turn-on?

A: I notice two things in your question that I want to address before I answer it. First, not all people get turned on by watching pornography. For some people, in fact, it's the exact opposite— a huge turn off. Other people really get turned on by watching pornography, and still others can take it or leave it. There's no "right" reaction. The important thing is to know what your own response is and why. Second, the phrase "watching pornography" is like the phrase "watching TV." It encompasses such a huge range of things that it's hard to think about as a whole. Just as there are different kinds of TV shows, of which some you'll like and others you won't, there are all different kinds of pornography. One kind might turn a person on while another doesn't. Now, for those people who are turned on by watching pornography, why is that? Again, there's no one right answer. Getting turned on can be a totally natural reaction to seeing something sexual, and it might be as simple as that. People who are visual learners (those who take in and process information more easily by seeing it than by hearing it) will likely be more turned on by viewing pornography than someone whose brain responds more to sounds or to physical movement. Some people create fantasies while watching pornography, which can be very stimulating, especially imagining that a sexual act they are seeing is being performed on them or by them. Fantasy is a normal way for our brains to try out ideas and doesn't necessarily have any connection to what we might actually do if given the opportunity in real life. Some people get turned on by doing something they think is "dirty," and if their value system says pornography is dirty, it might be the thrill of being "bad" that's the turn on. When people masturbate while watching pornography, they might associate watching the video with the physically stimulating sensations they are giving themselves; once the association is made, seeing the porn triggers the feelings.

Being turned on is a natural human response and can happen for a million different reasons. There's nothing inherently wrong with being turned on. As I said above, the more important question to think about is why and how it's happening, and whether that fits your values as an acceptable way to experience this very natural reaction.

Q: I've heard a lot of porn features orgies. What's an orgy? How many people can be in it?

A: An orgy is when a number of people all engage in sexual activity together. Orgies may be composed of people of any age, gender, sexual orientation, ability, etc. Couples can go to an orgy as well as single people. Some married or otherwise committed couples participate in orgies and some don't. Orgies rarely develop spontaneously (porn makes it seem like they do); they are almost always planned events where everyone who is going to it knows what's going to happen. Orgies can involve lots of switching of sexual partners. They aren't places where couples go who only want to have sex with each other. Some orgies have strict rules about everyone who is there using safer sex practices, and some don't. Some have guidelines to minimize the risk of sexual violence or assault happening, and some don't. While porn and popular media suggest orgies are no-risk, free-wheeling fun, that's seldom the truth. A person can experience both physical and emotional hurt if they're not careful. Many people find the idea of lots of people being sexual together to be immoral or wrong. As always, you have to know what your values are and be able to explain what you believe and why.

In terms of how many people are needed to make an orgy, there are no rules about that. We have a commonly used word for three people engaging in sexual activity together (a *threesome*), so I'd say the term *orgy* can apply when there's four or more people.

CHAPTER 10

Sexual Violence and Consent

Although Tarana Burke coined the phrase #MeToo in 2006, the movement exploded and gained global recognition in 2017. Communities were rocked by the barrage of reports from people of all genders, but especially women, speaking out about the sexual violence they experienced and continued to experience. A shift in consciousness was happening, not among those who had experienced violence, but for those who had never understood the scope of the problem before. Young people's voices were an important part of this movement, including at our school.

In 2017, a group of our twelfth-grade girls who had experienced various kinds of sexual harassment and violence gathered together to share stories and support one another. They also wanted to raise awareness in the school community that even here, in our seemingly safe and privileged "bubble," there were community members saying #MeToo.

The group gathered a long list of gender-based injustices they had experienced and wanted to bring it to their classmates. I feel compelled to say that the vast majority of the incidents on the list did not happen at school, but nevertheless they impacted how these students came to school, felt at school, and moved through their lives as students. Working with the school administration, a gathering of the twelfth-grade class was arranged. We met in a place that felt somewhat private, where we could all sit together in a circle and face one another. That turned out to be the wrestling room in the athletic center. We sat on the floor on the wrestling mats. The young women who planned the gathering randomly distributed the list of incidents they had collected to students who wished to participate in reading them aloud. We settled into silence, as is our practice as a Quaker school. Out of the silence came one voice after another sharing pain, hardship, injustice, fear, and anger. As the final voice finished, we returned to silence and reflection. There were quiet tears in the circle and when our time of reflection ended, students ran to hug, comfort, and console one another. Some students returned to their day. Others remained in the wrestling room seated on the mat sobbing with school counselors, teachers, and friends offering support.

Although this had been a meeting for the twelfth grade, of course, word spread through the rest of the high school. At our weekly Friday Student Council Assembly, a group of tenth-grade girls stood before the entire upper school and read a letter they had composed thanking their twelfth-grade sisters for speaking up. They felt protected and cared for by these older students, and their outpouring of sincere gratitude and love prompted more tears, although this time more happy and grateful than sad.

What Is Sexual Violence?

Sexual violence is difficult to talk about. It's not something we typically want to think about, and I can't imagine what a parent feels sending their beloved child out into a world where such violence exists. Yet because it exists we have to talk about it. We can't wait until kids are older to talk about this. The roots of sexual violence run deep; the seeds for it are planted long before adolescence. So, let's figure out how to talk about this in ways that are impactful, that align with our value systems, and that focus on information and skill development rather than fear.

The first thing I always do when talking about sexual violence is take the phrase #MeToo and invite students to consider a slightly altered version, #UsToo. We have plenty of available data that shows before kids turn eighteen, one in six boys and one in four girls will experience some form of sexual abuse. According to a 2021 article in *Pediatrics*, the journal of the American Academy of Pediatrics, 19 percent of transgender young people have experienced sexual abuse (and showed higher rates of psychological and physical abuse as well). So whenever we're in a group of people, we should assume there is someone there who is a survivor of, or is currently experiencing, sexual violence. That's a disturbing thought, but here's an even more disturbing one: for every person who experiences sexual violence, there's another person who perpetrates sexual violence. So, whenever we're in a group of people, we may also be in the presence of someone who has or is perpetrating sexual violence.

As kids look around the room, I always remind them that statistics are designed to address large groups. So, while they may not be accurate in our class of fifteen students, they get more accurate when you look at a high school of four hundred or one thousand or five thousand students. The point is, we have already encountered and will continue to encounter people who have experienced sexual violence, either as a survivor or as a perpetrator.

While it is true that there are certain groups that are more likely to experience sexual violence, for example women, trans people, and nonbinary people, there is no group or attribute that conveys complete immunity to sexual violence. It can happen to anyone; it can be perpetrated by anyone. At school that means remembering that sexual violence can happen in any of these ways: student perpetrator to student victim, adult perpetrator to student victim, student perpetrator to adult victim, and adult perpetrator to adult victim. Sexual violence can occur regardless of ability, age, ethnicity, gender, race, religion, sexual orientation, socioeconomic status, family structure, etc. This is something we all, no matter who we are, have to be informed about.

Let me say a quick word about the term *sexual violence*. I use this term deliberately to act as an umbrella that encompasses the many, many different kinds of behaviors that can occur when we talk about this topic. I use this graphic in class to illustrate this:

There are certainly terms in this list that students don't know, so we spend some time defining and talking about them. You may need to look up some as well. Students often ask why things like homophobia and misogyny/misandry are on the list. Those things aren't always physical; they can just be attitudes. That's true. Sexual violence doesn't just encompass the physical. It's an expression of violence that can be verbal, visual, physical, or digital. One's own, private thoughts and beliefs are not part of this. People are free to think and believe whatever they want. Once those beliefs or thoughts, if they are harmful to another person, get expressed in some way, that's when we need to pay attention.

Students also have a tendency to want to spend time focusing on some of the more extreme behaviors on the list. This allows me to raise a couple of important points. First, as extreme as they may seem, any of these behaviors can happen in one's community. Our school is situated in an affluent neighborhood just outside Philadelphia. We're on the Main Line, an area made famous in *The Philadelphia Story*. Yet even here, among large houses and manicured lawns, any of these things can and have happened. Second, I encourage students not to focus on the things that could *possibly* happen (which is all of them), but to think about the forms of sexual violence that are most *likely* to happen in their community, whether that's their neighborhood at home or here at school. The distinction between possible and likely is a very useful one. I use it when talking about all kinds of topics—everything from vulnerability to STIs to managing anxiety about tests.

Something that's possible might happen or it might not. We don't tend to spend a lot of time thinking about it, and while we can try to plan for it, it's not the best use of our energy. Yes, it's possible that as we sit in a classroom the ceiling can collapse, but I point out that none of the students are wearing football helmets or are holding little umbrellas over their heads à la Wile E. Coyote. (And then I have to explain Wile E. Coyote and the Road Runner, and I am reminded once again how old I am and how young they are.)

So, we go back to the list and I ask them to silently select three things that they think are likely to happen here at school. Later, in an anonymous evaluation of the class, I'll ask them to list the three things they selected. The data is remarkably similar year after year. Four things come up with disquieting regularity: homophobia, misogyny, unwanted sexting, and/or unwanted touching. Once we have this data, we can talk about how they happen, why they happen, and how we might work to prevent them.

Sexual Harassment, Sexual Assault, and Age of Consent Laws

Information is a crucial element in understanding and preventing sexual violence. I think every teen needs a clear understanding of sexual harassment, sexual assault, and how age of consent laws work. I cover these in detail in the tenth-grade health class and again in assemblies and other classes I provide at school.

A word of caution as I get into this. Laws about sexual harassment, assault, and age of consent vary by state. I live and work in Pennsylvania, so the information I have is based on the laws here. You should be sure to look up any particulars about these laws in your own state. While a lot of the general information will be the same, some things will be different. I am also not a lawyer, have had no legal training, and have no desire to be a lawyer. I claim no authority other than as an educator who has done my best to understand and communicate information about these topics clearly to students.

Sexual harassment is generally tied to a place: a school, a workplace, etc. It certainly can happen anywhere, but it's often talked about as site-specific. I talk with students about what it looks like in school. The definition I provide for sexual harassment in school comes from a professional development training our faculty received some years ago that was given by a legal professional. It is "unwelcome or unwanted physical, verbal, visual (including digital) behavior of a sexual nature that interferes with a person's school opportunities." That needs to be unpacked, so let's do that. The behavior has to be unwelcome or unwanted, however, this does not mean that a potential victim of sexual harassment has to say in advance all the behaviors they would consider such. Sexual harassment is a crime where *impact is more important than intent.* No matter what the potential perpetrator intended, if the victim finds it unwelcome or unwanted, it can count. Next, the behavior needs to be of a sexual nature. Remember, sexuality includes our bodies, our gender identity and expression, our sexual and romantic orientation, our actions, and our relationships. Unwelcome or unwanted behavior that is based on or impacts any of those aspects of a person counts, which means it can be physical, verbal, or visual (including digital). That covers a lot of ground, but note that it doesn't cover thought. Again, people are free to think and believe whatever they want. It's when that gets translated into action that we may have a problem. Here's another chart I use in class to explore some of the behaviors in these categories. This is not an exhaustive list, just some examples:

Sexual Harassment in School

Verbal: Sexual comments, slurs, teasing, jokes; sexual innu-endo; spreading sexual rumors about a person

Physical: Touching, grabbing, or pinching someone in a sexual way; intentionally brushing up against someone in a sexual way

Visual/Digital: Flashing, mooning; sexual gestures, looks, or leering; making or sharing sexual comments, images, or material online

The last part of the definition can be the trickiest. The behavior has to interfere with a student's ability to be at school or to perform in school as they wish. So, if you're having trouble concentrating in class because your phone keeps blowing up with unwanted sexts or sexual comments, that can count. If you have to change your route to get to math class, or you stay home from school altogether, because you want to avoid that student who always gets too "handsy" with you, that can count. If you can't study for a test because the kids at the next table in the library are making lewd comments about you, that can count. Again, impact takes precedence over intent. Sexual harassment happens in schools. Often it goes unreported to school officials, although students may discuss it among themselves. Talking with your teen about the kinds of behaviors listed above as potentially harassing can allow them to become a more observant member of their school community and hopefully to interrupt or prevent harassing behaviors from happening.

Sexual assault is a crime where intent does matter. The definition I use for this comes from the same faculty professional development training I mentioned above. It is "intentional sexual contact using force, threat, or abuse of power/authority, or when the victim does not or cannot consent." Most students find this definition clearer than the one for harassment. The definition uses the phrase *sexual contact*, which covers a wide array of behaviors, not limited to sexual intercourse. It's important to note that the threat of force is enough to make something qualify as sexual assault, even if no actual force is used. Also, we need to talk about what abuse of power or authority looks like. I start by asking kids what gives one student power or authority over another student. They quickly generate a long list: age, physical size or strength, sexual experience, social status, access to money, a driver's license, intellect, understanding the way the community works better than someone else does, good mental health, being a member of a majority group, etc. We can really quickly and easily fill the board with all the things that can potentially be used as power. If any of those things get used to force sexual activity to happen, it can count.

Most states don't just have one crime called sexual assault. There can be several different permutations depending on how the event happened, what kind of sexual contact occurred, and other factors like whether a weapon was involved in perpetrating the act. It's not important to memorize every possible version of sexual assault in your state, although as an adult you might want to know where to look for that information to help you answer questions your kids might have. Sexual assault can certainly happen at school, but it's more likely to happen at a party or some out-of-school event, especially where alcohol or other substances are being used and abused. Understanding the basics of sexual assault can help your teen protect themselves and their friends.

As you may know, teenagers can be pretty legalistic, and most of them don't want to get in trouble. They ask all kinds of questions about exactly where the lines are between harassment and assault and how alcohol or other substances impact whether one is culpable in a given situation, and they often ask about false reports.

I don't claim to have all the answers to their questions. Some we look up together during class, which can be a great lesson in determining what's a reliable source of information and what isn't. A college kid's blog isn't necessarily as useful as something from the American Bar Association. By doing a quick Google search the class learned that in our state, intoxication isn't an excuse to avoid prosecution for sexual assault, so even if both people are drunk, and even if the perpetrator was so drunk they don't remember assaulting the victim, they can still be held accountable if the evidence points to it. That was a sobering (no pun intended) moment for a lot of my kids who assumed that if both people were drunk it was a "no harm, no foul" situation. We also discovered that in our state if a perpetrator uses alcohol to incapacitate a potential victim, the severity of the crime they can be charged with increases. Having kids look up this information, or looking it up with them, can be more impactful than just telling them.

Remember, this really isn't a lesson or a conversation about legalities. It's raising awareness of some specific kinds of sexual violence that we don't want any teen to have to deal with, as a victim or as a perpetrator.

Questions about age of consent laws often arise during these conversations. I find these laws are very often misunderstood by teens. The age of consent is how old a person must be *legally* to consent to having sexual activity with another person. Each state sets their own age of consent and can also add exceptions to this law. If a person over the age of consent has sexual activity with a person under the age of consent, the older person can be charged with a crime called statutory rape. In Pennsylvania, where my school is located, the age of consent is sixteen. That means that anyone under the age of sixteen cannot legally consent to sex with any other person no matter what age. So, if a person aged sixteen years or older engages in sexual activity with someone who is under the age of sixteen, the sex is considered illegal because the younger person does not have the legal capacity to say yes to it.

Remember, though, I said states can also modify these laws if they choose. Pennsylvania has something commonly called a "Romeo and Juliet" clause. It says that if the younger person in the interaction is between the ages of thirteen and fifteen, and the older person is no more than four years older than the younger person, the older person will not *necessarily* be charged with statutory rape if the sexual relationship comes to light. This modification recognizes that in some circumstances relationships between younger and older teenagers happen and the crime of statutory rape may not be appropriate in all these instances. (By the way, I'm not saying I'm in favor of this modification, just that it exists.)

The sexual activity still *can* be considered statutory rape but it doesn't automatically *have* to be. An encounter between an older and younger teen or between two kids under the age of consent may still be a case of sexual assault. It's just the one, specific crime of statutory rape that *may* not apply. It's not a "get out of jail free card."

If, however, my students go to New York for the weekend, they need to know that New York's age of consent is sixteen and there are no exceptions or modifications granted. One of the activities I do with my twelfth-graders each year is to look up the age of consent laws in the states where they plan to attend college. This is essential information that any young person should know. We also look up each school's policy on sexual harassment, sexual assault, and any other policies regarding sexual activity and consent that a school may have. You should do this with your teen not only for college, but for places they go on vacation, or summer camps they may go to outside of your state of residence. It can be especially enlightening to look at the laws in other countries they may travel to for exchange trips or semesters abroad.

All this legal information may have your head spinning. Remember, this is just information. The idea is to get kids talking about these issues so that they can avoid problems. Again, don't be accusatory. Be informative and open, welcome questions, and work together to find the information needed to make your kid smart and savvy about these issues.

The Roots of Sexual Violence

One of the most important things to consider about sexual violence is that it doesn't just appear out of nowhere. A person is much more likely to be harassed or assaulted by someone they know than by a stranger. When looking at a community where sexual harassment or assault has become an issue, it is clear that long before these horrible acts were committed, there were other beliefs and practices alive in the community that made the events more possible, or even more likely.

Several years ago, I attended a lecture by Dr. Jackson Katz. If you don't know about him or his work, I urge you to visit his website (https://www.jacksonkatz.com/). Katz is a speaker, author, and researcher. His work has been to examine the roots of gender-based violence and work to promote gender equity. His TED Talk, "Violence Against Women—It's a Men's Issue," has over two and a half million views. Katz is an expert in working with men to help them understand and accept their role in gender-based violence, and he does so with great tact and sensitivity. He doesn't berate men; rather he allies himself with them to help them see that such violence can be as damaging to them as it is to the women who suffer it.

In the lecture I saw, Katz asked the audience to imagine a pyramid (a triangle) with several horizontal lines creating different levels moving up the triangle. If you go to Google Images and type in "pyramids of sexual violence" you will see many different versions of these pyramids. At the top of the pyramid, at the narrowest point, is where the most egregious examples of sexual violence live, things like rape, incest, "crimes of passion," etc. At each level below on the pyramid are forms of lesser, but no less horrible, violence that, if left unaddressed, set the stage for the violence above it to take place. This can be anything from sexual harassment, to catcalling (now often called street harassment), to inequity in pay based solely on gender, to unwanted sexting, to humor that degrades women or LGBTQIA+ people. If a person or a community is only paying attention to the very top of the pyramid, they're taking an entirely reactive stance to sexual violence. They're only acting after some horrible event has already taken place. The time to start thinking about sexual violence isn't after we hear of a person who was assaulted at a party, or after a survivor tells their story as a participant in a panel at a school assembly.

Where Katz asked the audience to focus was on the very bottom of the pyramid. This was an area where he labeled unexamined ideas, standard practices, and cultural assumptions. Here, Katz argued, are the true roots of sexual violence. They're in what we're leaving unexamined every day in our life or in the life of a community we inhabit. For example, a community that runs on a "boys will be boys" attitude, or an individual who sees no problem telling jokes about rape or assault, or a school that normalizes gender inequity rather than gender equity. Any of these things can create an atmosphere where more serious kinds of sexual violence can occur. Katz argued these things can be hard to see because they are so normalized that they are seemingly invisible without deliberate effort to notice them. When we focus attention on this level of the pyramid, we become more proactive in preventing and interrupting sexual violence. By preventing lesser kinds of sexual violence we can help stop larger incidences from happening. Here's an example from my own school's history about something that lived for a long time at the bottom of our pyramid.

The walls along the majestic wooden stairway of our Main Building are lined with photos of graduating classes going back decades. In the vast majority of the photos, girls and boys are separated, girls on the left and boys on the right, or boys in the back and girls in the front. The girls are wearing white dresses and the boys are wearing dark suits. The photos are lovely. The graduates are beaming, and current students love to scour the photos to find their parents, older siblings, grandparents, and even some current faculty members who are graduates of the school. Many, many independent schools have the tradition of wearing some kind of formal attire at graduation that is often segregated by gender. This is simply the way graduation is done. It's a time-honored tradition. Oh, there were occasional comments through the years about it being "old-fashioned" or even sexist, but it was never *really* a problem, until we saw it in a different light.

Our school prides itself on being open to all, and that includes embracing and honoring our transgender and gender nonconforming students for whom our graduation tradition was problematic, even painful. It took a process of education, deep conversation, deeper listening, a few missteps, and affirming our commitment to who we wanted to be as a school that led to a change. Now our students graduate in identical caps and gowns, and the class sits alphabetically on the stage rather than in gendered groups. Kids assert their individuality by decorating their mortarboard caps in all kinds of fun and wonderful ways. At the base of the stairs in the Main Building are the photos of the most recent graduating classes in their caps and gowns. What once seemed like an unthinkable change became something we couldn't not change. The world kept spinning and the school kept moving forward, as one unexamined idea got removed from the bottom of our pyramid.

You can certainly think about your own child's school and what might lie at the bottom of their pyramid, but I'd also urge you to examine your own family's values, beliefs, and practices— your own family pyramid. Might you see something that, without intending to, might contribute to your child becoming more vulnerable to sexual violence either as a victim or a perpetrator? What might that conversation look like with your child or with your family? Remember, the goal is to interrupt and prevent sexual violence, to keep kids safe and whole, and to help them avoid some of the ugliest experiences life can contain. That's worth the work of noticing what may have gone unnoticed so far, isn't it?

Consent: The Antidote to Sexual Violence

This chapter is a heavy one, and I don't want you to think there's no solution to the problem of sexual violence. There is, and it's deceptively simple: it's understanding and grounding ourselves in *consent*. Every incidence of sexual violence begins as a violation of someone's consent. No one intentionally seeks out or welcomes sexual violence into their lives. It's an intrusion and a violation, and given the chance, I don't know anyone who wouldn't say "No thank you" to it.

I've talked about consent in my Sexuality and Society classes over the years, and the responses from the students have always been curious to me. They clearly understand that when it comes to initiating sexual activity with another person, whether with a hookup or with a sweetheart, consent is absolutely essential. No one argues with that. The problem comes with how to establish consent.

"You mean I actually have to ask someone whether I can kiss them or not?" a boy in a preppy polo asks.

"Uh, yeah," replies a black-haired, heavily mascaraed boy with ear piercings and multicolored fingernails. "You can't just walk up to someone and put your tongue down their throat."

"No, of course. That's not what I mean," the preppy boy snaps back, "but do I have to actually say it with words? I mean, body language can say it for you."

"We've talked about different kinds of communication," I interject, "and we've established that nonverbal communication is perfectly valid, and often perfectly imperfect."

"Well, except for sign language, right?" a red-haired girl who's a bit of a smart aleck says. "You wouldn't say ASL is perfectly imperfect, would you, Mr. V?"

"No, I wouldn't say that." I sigh, showing more exasperation than I'd like to. "And let's not get sidetracked talking about ASL, OK?"

When it comes to verbally assessing sexual consent, my students always find they face the word, and the feeling, they dread the most.

"It's just so *AWKWARD*!" they practically scream in unison.

Awkward is kryptonite to adolescents. It saps their will and makes them weak and pliable. They'll do almost anything to avoid looking or feeling awkward. I get it, adolescence is a time of building agency and identity. It's about mastering skills and successfully navigating experiences. No one wants to be the awkward kid. The irony is, the only way to conquer awkwardness is to walk through it and come out the other end. Kids who spend their teenage years trying to avoid awkward situations never conquer them and grow up to become adults who never learn how to deal with awkward situations.

I've made a mantra out of the phrase "Life is awkward!" in all my classes. I say it so often that even I get bored of saying it. I'm also known for saying that the only thing more awkward than talking about having sex with someone is actually having sex with someone.

"It's not like the movies, or porn! People get cramps. People fart. People roll off the bed or onto someone's hair, or their arm gets trapped underneath someone. It's fumbly and funny and sweaty and sometimes it's romantic and passionate and wonderful, but even then it's still awkward!"

"You're not doing it right," a voice says quietly from the back of the room. I let that go unanswered. It's a trap; there's no good response. I just smile and move on.

I've tried different activities to get students to practice negotiating sexual consent. We've used random snippets of conversation to create dialogues, with the outcome of agreeing to have sex and not agreeing to have sex. We've tried to find good media examples of conversations about sexual consent (it's harder than it seems). We've tried creating conversations about consent where the topic isn't negotiating sex. And that's where I had my Aha! moment. Being in my class helps students talk freely and openly about sex.

That's not the awkward part for them. It's the negotiation, the very act of asking someone for something, or inviting them into an experience that feels daunting. I wondered why that might be, and the conclusion I've come to is that we're not doing a good enough job highlighting the everyday consent experiences in our lives. So, I had to find a new way to teach about consent, and I had to help my students see that they're already quite skilled in negotiating consent; they just don't know that they are. So, here's my new approach to talking about consent, and I offer it to you to use with your own kids.

Of course, the first thing we need to start with is a definition. If kids of any age need help defining what exactly consent is, the easiest definition is that it's *asking permission to do something or inviting someone to do something.* Consent is linked to an action. You don't need consent to think something about someone else, but you always need consent to do something to or with someone else. Consent always has two parts, the invitation and the response. Both are essential. With little kids I compare it to a birthday party invitation. If you invite someone to come to your birthday party and they never respond, how do you know what to do next? How many chairs should you set up? How many goodie bags do you need? How much cake do you need to make sure everyone has a yummy piece? I did a talk at a college once and afterward a young man approached me with a question. He was pursuing a young woman he really liked. He had asked her out a couple of times and she politely declined. He wanted to know what to do next.

"Nothing," I said. "She's given you her answer."

"But shouldn't I keep trying?" he asked earnestly. "I really want to go out with her."

"You asked. She answered. That's it," I said. "If you continue to ask, you're just badgering her and that's creepy and wrong."

"But she didn't even give me a reason. She just said no."

"She doesn't have to give you a reason. You asked. She answered," I repeated. This young man wasn't a creep or a sexual predator; he just didn't understand the basics of consent.

In order to get students of any age to understand how ubiquitous consent is, I tell them that whenever we interact with another person's *body*, *property*, or *reputation* we need to obtain consent. Think about how many times a day you interact with someone else's body, property, or reputation. Given the number of times this happens, we should all be experts in practicing and negotiating consent, but we're not. So why not? Is it because we're not actually seeking consent in these interactions? Are we assuming we have consent without checking it out to be sure? Are we just callous brutes who don't care about other people at all? It's probably not that. What if we could become more conscious of these consent situations and were more deliberate about establishing consent in them? How would our world change? How would the larger society change? And how would our interactions specifically about sexual consent change? I really believe if we were better at practicing everyday consent, establishing sexual consent would seem much more natural and easy.

I've had the chance to meet some pretty amazing people in my work. A couple of summers ago, I was a guest on a podcast hosted by Katie Couric. I was a little starstruck to be honest and I really wanted to take a photo with her. She was completely gracious about it. When I approached her, I asked, as has become my custom (I practice what I preach), "Is it OK if I put my arm around your shoulder in the photo?" She paused for a moment and then smiled and said, "Sure." I'm sure she takes a million photos with fans. I wonder how many actually ask before putting their arms around her? I'm not any kind of hero for doing that. I'm just someone who has become very conscious of my everyday interactions and I work really hard to practice everyday consent.

Engage your child about all the different ways they interact with someone else's body in a given day, and see how many of those times they deliberately established consent. This isn't a "gotcha!" question. I believe people do actually practice body consent a lot; they just aren't conscious of it. A lot of consent around body-to-body interactions is nonverbal. Someone raises a hand for a high-five and you respond. The hand raising of the first person is an invitation, a nonverbal request to interact with your body. You either do or don't high-five back.

OK, now think about touching somebody else's body accidentally—maybe you bump into someone at the store. Typically we apologize. Why? Because we initiated some kind of body contact without consent. It was an accident, not an assault, but our reflex is to apologize. If we don't acknowledge the accident, sometimes the other person gets annoyed or even angry. Why? Because there's been a violation of their bodily autonomy, and we expect people, especially strangers, to ask before touching us.

Interacting with other people's property may be even more commonplace than interacting with bodies. One of the things that really annoys me is when I see a student pick up some other kid's cell phone and start diddling with it. The only time I touch my husband's cell phone is if I think he's left it somewhere accidentally and I want to bring it to him. I certainly have never swiped through any of his apps or texts anything like that. Yet my students don't seem to think about consent at all when it comes to other people's devices. They'll ask to borrow a pen before just taking one, but they'll change a friend's ringtone or home screen photo "as a joke." Ugh! A more common property consent violation has probably happened to you or your kid around food. Perhaps you've ordered a delicious plate of fries only to have a friend reach across, grab one off your plate, and as they're bringing the fry to their mouth they ask, "Can I have a fry?" What are you supposed to say? If you say no, are they supposed to put it back on your plate? Eww!

Bodies and property are pretty easy to understand, so now let's talk about reputation a bit. Your reputation is how other people see you or what other people think about you. It's the echo of you that lives on after your physical presence is gone. One of the artifacts of the digital world is that it's super easy to talk about people without them ever knowing what we're saying about them. We see a post about someone we know and we share it or retweet it, but how often do we check in with the person to make sure they're OK with that information about them being shared? The same thing happened before the digital world existed. You heard something about someone and you passed it on without checking it out. Remember what we called that? It was gossip or a rumor, and it wasn't considered very polite. People should be able to have some control over their reputations. One of the ways that happens is if others seek consent before sharing information about us.

An exercise you can do with your teen is to pick one of the areas of everyday consent (body, property, or reputation) and ask them to try to be especially mindful about it for a week. Make a chart on the fridge like you did when they were little to track each day whether they were mostly successful or mostly unsuccessful in practicing consent in that area. Talk with them about it in the evening, encourage them, and listen when they tell you about successes and struggles. This is about becoming more deliberate, not about becoming perfect. I loathe the phrase "Practice makes perfect." I prefer "Practice makes progress." Any step we help young people take in becoming more conscious and skilled in everyday consent will help them in the long run, including in negotiating sexual consent.

When talking about sexual consent with my students, one of the things that raises the awkward flag is having to be honest with someone else about what they do or don't want sexually. Telling a sexual partner that they're not getting you off is never fun, but it's honest. One of the things we can stress when talking with kids about everyday consent is that it also brings a great opportunity to practice being honest in situations that aren't as fraught as sexual activity. In fact, for consent to be valid, honesty has to be part of it. The person asking for consent has to be honest (and specific) about what they do or don't want. It's not honest to ask to touch someone's arm if you really want to touch their breast. It's not honest to ask to *borrow* a pencil if you have no intention of returning it. On the other side, the person responding to the consent request or invitation has to say yes when they mean yes, no when they mean no, and maybe when they mean maybe. This can be especially difficult in our "post-truth" society, but it's a skill we have to practice and maintain. Life just goes so much more smoothly when we can trust what people say to us.

In a class of tenth-graders, I pose this question: "How many of you have been in a situation, not necessarily a sexual situation—

any kind of situation—where you said yes when you meant no? Raise your hand if you have." Lots of hands go up. "Why do we do this?" I turn to write on the board as they shout out answers.

"You don't want to hurt someone's feelings."

"It's just easier to say yes than to say no."

"You're afraid to say no."

"You don't really care either way."

"You don't really have a choice. They just make it look like you do."

This interaction allows me to bring up another important point about consent. Power disrupts and can even negate consent. Consent is only valid when we actually have the chance to say yes or no. If we're afraid or feeling pressured, or if for any reason we can't respond honestly, consent isn't valid. In the case of sexual activity, that can bring us right back to sexual harassment and assault like we talked about earlier in the chapter.

Other things that can cause consent to fail include: dishonesty on the part of the person asking for consent, a genuine misunderstanding of what's being negotiated, not being able to think clearly, perhaps because one's mind is clouded by alcohol or drugs, or lack of knowledge about what's happening. We can easily imagine any of these things happening. Again, we're not seeking perfection. We're trying to practice better everyday consent in the service of establishing better consent around sexual situations.

I've mentioned nonverbal consent earlier in this chapter. Just to clarify, consent can successfully be given nonverbally. I always add these caveats when talking to kids, though: verbal consent is always preferable to nonverbal consent, and the more serious the matter is, the more verbal consent is important. There's a reason when you're seated in the exit row of an airplane the flight attendant has to actually hear you say "yes" when they ask if you're able to follow the emergency procedures in the event of a problem. That's too important a situation not to have the clearest answer possible. If you want to interact sexually with someone else's body, it's certainly better to have an enthusiastic verbal response than a shrug. And speaking of shrugs: silence, noncommittal reactions, and a verbal or nonverbal "no" do not convey consent. Also, prior consent for something does not convey consent for a new situation.

Consent, whether it's around everyday body, property, or reputation interactions or sexual interactions, should be affirmative, enthusiastic, honest, revocable, and situation specific. So, say it loud and proud—YES!!

....

Question Box:

Q: Why is sex an uncomfortable topic to talk about? Since it is an especially uncomfortable topic for most people in the United States, what factors are unique to the United States that make it that way?

A: As we noted in class, the US compares quite poorly to European nations when looking at things like rate of teenage pregnancy, abortion rates, STD rates among young people, rates of sexual assault, and other factors. It's easy to assume that the Puritan ideas of the first US settlers set the stage for our general anxiety about sex, but that doesn't hold up to scrutiny. The

Puritans were just as interested in sex as anyone else (in fact, they were kinda kinky in some ways). There are a number of factors that combine to make our nation less open to talking about sexuality. It might be the large amount of people who belong to religious organizations that have generally negative or sinful views of sexuality. It might be that sexual freedom and equality are not thought of as fundamental rights in our Constitution or laws. It could be related to politics and using fear and stigma about sex to gain political favor with voters. There isn't any one reason.

In general, we seemed to be trending toward more openness, but we're now seeing a large pushback in the proliferation of anti-trans and "don't say gay" laws currently being introduced in state legislatures and the overturning of Roe v. Wade. Being able to communicate openly and honestly about sex and working toward sexual justice are things we have to work towards deliberately. They won't just happen by themselves.

Q: How do you best handle a situation where you or someone you know is falsely accused of sexual harassment or sexual assault?

AND

Q: What should you do if mutual consent is clearly given for a sexual encounter where you are one of the people involved, but later, the other person untruthfully says that they did not give consent for the purpose of getting you punished?

A: First of all (and this is not addressing these specific questions above—I'll do that in a minute) creating a false account of sexual assault is rare. Of all the accusations made about sexual assault or consent violations, experts estimate somewhere between 2 percent and 10 percent of accusations are false. *That means that 90 to 98 percent of accusations are true. So, believing people who bring forth accusations of sexual assault or harassment is essential.*

Now, to these specific questions. The best way to fend off a false allegation is to be able to provide clear, concrete evidence that the incident didn't happen, or didn't happen in the way it's being described. Was anyone else there who can corroborate your side of the story? Is anyone willing to come forward to say they heard the accuser say they were making a false allegation to punish someone? Can the person being accused provide evidence of conversations they had with other people about the alleged event? For example, maybe they talked with a friend about how they did establish consent in the situation. Has this person ever been accused of sexual misconduct before? Does the pattern of their past actions suggest this accusation is out of character for them? If it comes down to one person's word against another, that's a very difficult situation to sort out. It's important that a person who feels they are being falsely accused talk to an adult or someone in authority who can help them.

Q: A longtime friend of mine is expressing some very concerning ideas about sex and sexuality. I talked to a friend of his and she said that he's made some advances on her and has been getting increasingly angry at her and her friends. He also described wanting a woman to be "silent and still" during intercourse. What can I do to ensure that myself and my friends stay safe/how do I talk to him about this without setting him off?

A: I can see how this would be troubling, and I appreciate your desire both to be safe and to help your friend confront these harmful ideas. You should not put yourself in danger. Walk away from the situation if you have any fears about your own mental or physical safety. If you do choose to engage, clear communication and drawing firm boundaries are very important when dealing with someone who is expressing thoughts like these. It's important for your female friend to be clear that his advances and his anger are not welcome and that if they persist, she will have to involve someone like his folks at home or an adult in the school community to make them stop. She can also decide to sever contact completely with him if she thinks that would be best for her own safety or mental health. In terms of talking with your friend without "setting him off," unfortunately there's no way to guarantee that. He sounds like he might be influenced by misogynist ideas. These are very dangerous ideas and he needs to understand how out of step they are both rationally and morally.

It's not your job to fix your friend, but you certainly can invite him to talk to a counselor or therapist about how he's feeling. You also need to set firm boundaries with him about what you're willing to talk about, and let him know that your friendship may be threatened if he persists in these ideas. *And this last piece is important: if he expresses ideas about hurting himself or other people, don't wait—contact an adult immediately and report what you heard.*

Epilogue

The changes I see in my students as they move through my Sexuality and Society class are amazing. At the outset, they're giggly, nervous, a bit defensive, and generally pretty confused about sexuality. By the time they leave the class, they're confident, open, and more secure in themselves, and they know their values. I'm not a miracle worker, and I don't know some great secret that their parents don't know. I simply talk to them.

I want to wrap up, not with more of my words—you've had enough of them—but with some of their words. Near the end of the course, I give out blank index cards to the kids and ask them to write down some words of wisdom they learned in our class that they want to pass on to the ninth-graders in our school. I tell them this is their chance to be the "sexperts," to give the younger members of our community the benefit of *their* wisdom. They take this task very seriously; they really *do* care about the younger kids, and the legacy they're leaving for them. I have to admit to getting a little weepy when I read through the index cards. Here's what they had to say:

"No one is normal. No one. I mean it, no one. Yet people will still try to pretend they are all the same in every way. Everyone who does this is lying in some manner, and will be much happier when they find the self-confidence to stop."

"Whether you hooked up with them, broke up with them, went out with them, or did anything else with them, remember their feelings matter too. Getting hurt sucks when it happens to you; don't do it to them just to satisfy your pride. They'll remember just like you do."

"Just 'cause it's available doesn't mean you should do it! Pursue things that you actively want to pursue."

"Don't rely on the love of others to make yourself feel loved. Love yourself first."

"Keep an open mind, but know your own opinions. Be strong in who you are."

"If you have anything holding you back from sex, don't have sex. It should be something that stems from complete body and soul 'Yes!'"

"Don't be embarrassed to talk to people, friends, sweethearts, parents. The more you talk about anything and everything, the better you will be."

"You don't need to fit a label, whether that label is straight, gay, bisexual, artist, athlete, or anything else."

"It's not your body that determines how attracted people are to you. It's how you feel about your body."

"Pay attention to double standards."

"Saying 'no pressure' and 'no expectations' often means the opposite."

"It's OK to have sex. You're not a bad person if you do."

"During high school people might try to make you feel as though you have to be in a relationship because that's what's 'supposed to happen' in high school. Just make sure you know: it's OK to want to be or to be in a committed relationship. It's OK not to want to be or not to be in a committed relationship. It's OK to just be single."

"Your first time having sex is never going to live up to the hype/buildup. Whether it's awesome or uncomfortable, think of it as a learning experience rather than the most sexual act of your life."

"Everything is easier when you communicate. No one can read your mind so you have to put what you want out there. Aside from that, the most important thing is listening. You can learn a lot by listening in all aspects of life, especially sex."

"Your friends are going through the same things you are, probably have similar questions, so seek them out and seek out educators so you can become knowledgeable and help not only yourself but others as well."

"You don't need to be in a relationship to be cool. You don't need to do anything sexual to be cool. If you can't talk about what you want to do, don't do it."

"Don't use sex to try to climb the social ladder."

"It's OK to be confused, to be complicated, to be scared, to make mistakes; it will all be OK, and it is most definitely OK to be you—whoever and whatever you are."

Does this sound good to you? Do you wish your own child would say, or believe, or act according to these ideas? The good news is, they can, and they certainly don't have to take my class. *You* can help facilitate the same changes in the young people who live under your roof. Give them the chance to talk without fear of being judged. Give them permission to ask questions, seek answers, make decisions, and make mistakes. Help them to filter out, or at least recognize, external expectations and hold those expectations up to what they've discovered to be their authentic selves. See, none of this is about being a sex expert or knowing everything there is to know about sex. It's all about the relationship, the interaction, and the openness to say, "Let's talk."

Good luck.

Acknowledgments

I'll never write a book!" was my constant refrain whenever my friend Trish suggested it. Perhaps I was hesitant because I imagined writing a book to be a solitary process—just me, my thoughts, and a blank page. What could be more terrifying or daunting? What I've learned, though, is that writing a book, at least writing *this* book, has been a wonderfully communal experience. It does take a village, and I am grateful and honored to have shared this work with so many extraordinary people:

First and foremost, many thanks to Brooke Lea Foster for her invaluable assistance in preparing this book's original manuscript.

Thanks to Scott Waxman at Waxman Leavell Literary Agency, to Gabrielle Sellei at Semanoff, Ormsby, Greenberg, and Torchia, and to Julie Will and Emma Kupor at HarperCollins for believing in me and shepherding me through this process.

Thanks to Albert Angelo, Liza Ewen, Laurie Novo, and Jordan Taffet, who read early drafts of this manuscript and provided loving, helpful, and wise feedback.

Thanks to the Friends' Central community: administrators, faculty, staff, and students who continually encouraged me, supported me, and celebrated my successes with me.

Thanks to the community of professional sexuality educators, especially the members of ASET (Advanced Sexuality Educators and Trainers) who have been my personal and professional mentors, colleagues, confidants, and friends.

Thanks to my family of choice, especially: Trish, Eric, Todd, Jeanmarie, Margaret, Jay, and Mr. Nelson, for sticking with me through thick and thin.

And finally, thanks to my dear husband, Michael, for . . . well, for everything.

This is my village. I love them one and all.

Index

About the Author

Al Vernacchio is a high school sexuality educator and English teacher at Friends' Central School in Wynnewood, Pennsylvania. In addition to his classroom responsibilities, Al organizes sexuality-themed programs and assemblies, provides parent education on human sexuality topics, and is one of the faculty advisors for the Gay-Straight Alliance. A human sexuality educator and consultant for more than twenty-five years, Al Vernacchio has lectured, published articles, and offered workshops throughout the country. His work has been featured in "Teaching Good Sex," a November 20, 2011, cover story in the *New York Times Magazine*. Al has given four TED Talks and has appeared on national programs such as NPR's *Morning Edition* and *1A*. Al earned his BA in theology from St. Joseph's University and his MSEd in human sexuality education from the University of Pennsylvania. He is a member of the Society for the Scientific Study of Sexuality (SSSS); the American Association of Sexuality Educators, Counselors, and Therapists (AASECT); and Advanced Sexuality Educators and Trainers (ASET). A lifelong Philadelphian, Al and his husband, Michael, live in the Germantown section of the city.